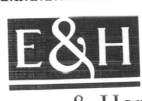

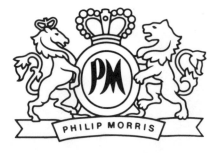

HEALTH FACT, HEALTH FICTION

▸ ▸ ▸ ▸ ▸ ▸ ▸ ▸ ▸ ▸ ▸ ▸ ▸ ▸ ▸ ▸ ▸ ▸ ▸

Getting Through the Media Maze

HEALTH FACT, HEALTH FICTION

▸ ▸

Getting Through the Media Maze

ROBERT L. TAYLOR, M.D.

Taylor Publishing Company ▸ ▸ ▸ Dallas, Texas

Published by Taylor Publishing Company,
  1550 West Mockingbird Lane,
  Dallas, Texas 75235
Design by Barbara E. Williams

Library of Congress Cataloging-in-Publication Data

Taylor, Robert L., 1942–
  Health fact, health fiction : getting through the
media maze / Robert L. Taylor.
      p.   cm.
    ISBN 0-87833-683-4 : $16.95
   1. Mass media in health education—United
States.   2. Health promotion—United States.
3. Advertising—Medicine—United States.
4. Health behavior.   5. Consumer education—
United States.   I. Title.
RA440.5.T39   1990
613′.0973—dc20   89-34579
                                                CIP

ISBN: 0-087833-683-4

Printed in the United States of America

10   9   8   7   6   5   4   3   2   1

To
Chuck Roppel
and
Fuller Torrey

ACKNOWLEDGMENTS

▸ ▸ ▸ ▸ ▸ ▸ ▸ ▸ ▸ ▸ ▸

I am grateful to several people who helped me conceive and write this book. David Lam, as he has so often in the past, discussed and countered some of my early thoughts.

Eugene Robin, Elizabeth Whelan, Leonard Syme, and John Urquhard shared their provocative ideas.

Elaine Patterson provided logistical support. Lisa Hunter, Mel Walsh, and Susan Beutler slogged through early drafts and gave me the good news and the bad news.

June Flora argued with me. The book is better for it. Marjorie Kwawer watched over the early manuscript. Melinda Mossar supportively read and commented.

Corinne Wilburne raised thoughtful questions and reviewed the final manuscript.

Finally, I want to thank Bob Sehlinger for pushing just hard enough and Stevie Henderson and Barbara Williams for their wonderful editing touches.

▸ ▸ ▸ ▸ ▸

Be careful about reading health books; you may die of
a misprint.

Mark Twain

CONTENTS

▸ ▸ ▸ ▸ ▸ ▸

HEALTH FACT, HEALTH FICTION

▸ ▸ ▸ ▸ ▸ ▸ ▸ ▸ ▸ ▸ ▸ ▸ ▸ ▸ ▸ ▸ ▸ ▸ ▸ ▸

Getting Through the Media Maze

▸ ▸ ▸ ▸ ▸

DR. MELIK: You mean there was no deep fat? No steak or cream pies? Or hot fudge?

DR. TYRON [smugly]: Those were thought to be un-healthy—exactly the opposite of what we now know to be true.

[Exchange between two scientists looking back on twentieth-century health beliefs]

—from the film *Sleeper,*
Woody Allen

WARNING: THE VERY ACT OF LIVING IS KNOWN TO BE DANGER-OUS TO HEALTH

—editorial, *Los Angeles Times,*
August 14, 1988

CHAPTER ONE

▸ ▸ ▸ ▸ ▸ ▸ ▸ ▸

Health Dread

If you fed into a computer all of the "medical breakthrough" head-lines and the special health reports that barrage you daily, and programmed the computer to collate this glut of information into a formula you could follow for a longer, healthier life, likely, it would self-destruct. And not just because it had been given an "information overload." The more probable cause would be that, time after time, the computer would find major discrepancies in the various reports.

That's why you should take all the health risks, health tips, and medical breakthroughs with a grain of salt—or a proverbial grain of salt if you believe all the bad press it's been getting (and you shouldn't). Actually, we're living longer, healthier lives today than ever before, yet much of what we hear is health hazard after health hazard, until it seems as if no matter what we do, we're putting our very lives at stake, daily.

Everything Is Bad for Us

In a sense, we should be thankful for the flood of health "facts." After all, at least we know enough to try to fight back. But where do we start? There are so many health hazards. How can we tell a big risk from a not-so-big risk? Perspective is hard to come by. Headlines don't discriminate. They are just as big for trivial health matters as they are for the most serious threats. It seems that everything is bad for us. We are left with the choice of either throwing up our hands in overwhelming frustration and living as if none of these health dangers really matters, or slowly obsessing ourselves into a state of total health dread.

Fat is bad. So is sitting around. Fast food is bad—all that salt and sugar. And forget ice cream; it's the kiss of death. Stress is bad. Smoking is bad. Being overweight is bad. The list goes on and on.

Book titles tell it all: *Eating May Be Hazardous to Your Health*, *Who's Poisoning America?*, and *Killer Salt*. Newspaper headlines and television commentaries are even worse: "Defusing Cancer's Timebomb," "The Politics of Poison," "Cholesterol Is Proved Deadly," "Coffee Causes Cancer." As if that were not bad enough, the story keeps changing.

In a frustrated letter to the *Los Angeles Times* (January 17, 1986), Edna McHugh, a resident of Malibu, California, summed up what a lot of us are feeling these days: "They're scaring us to death. 'Don't touch that drink!' 'Don't eat that hot dog!' 'Put out that cigarette!' 'Don't breathe.' There's a difference between information and bombardment. Twenty-four hours a day we are told that everything is killing us. Maybe it is, but so is fear."

Health dread is difficult to live with, but confused health dread is even worse. When *Newsweek*'s Meg Greenfield talks about how "nothing lasts," we all know exactly what she means. "No assertion has a shelf life of more than eleven months. . . . what is banned today is likely to be administered intravenously in all the best clinics tomorrow."

In his book *Making Health Decisions*, Dr. Thomas Vogt describes one of his heart patients who finally had had all he could take of talk about health risks. "What's the use?" he questioned. "These days it seems like everything is bad for you. It's not worth living in a closet to reach ninety. Everything you eat causes cancer, and everything else you enjoy causes heart disease. What's the point in trying to change anything?" Having gotten this off his chest, the patient put on his hat and left. Later, alone in his office, Dr. Vogt recalled his patient's frustration and jotted down all the alleged risk factors for heart disease he could think of. In a few minutes he had a list of thirty-eight items. He began to see his patient's point. It was pretty confusing. (In 1981, researchers James McCormick and Petr Skrabanek put together a list of 246 "risk factors" for coronary heart disease. The list continues to grow and now includes taking siestas, snoring, having English as a mother tongue, and not eating mackerel!)

This year's salt often turns out to be next year's broccoli. Or vice versa. It makes health dread that much more difficult to deal with. We feel we are never playing with a full deck. We can't believe what we are told, but we have to believe something. There's a lot riding on it.

There's no doubt about it; deciding what is and what is not healthy has become a full-time job. Ellen Goodman, the popular syndicated columnist, described it this way:

> I'm not sure whether to be grateful for these accumulated pieces of knowledge. What have I learned? Run too little and die young of a heart attack? Run too much and die, without offspring, of some bizarre infection? Drink your way to breast cancer? Abstain all the way to the coronary unit?
>
> I think it has become impossible for Americans to keep their health IQ updated. We are all suffering from an information glut, research overload. But worse, we have accumulated a midriff bulge of confusing and contradictory health advice.

Goodman is right. And the bias of the conflicting health news is negative. The world around us appears ominous, containing more health risks than benefits.

Different Slant

But there's another side to the story that receives far less attention than the health reports of doom and gloom. In a *Wall Street Journal* article entitled "Living Longer and Feeling Worse About It," the executive director of the American Council on Science and Health, Elizabeth Whelan, lays out some interesting facts. In 1900, newborns in this country lived an average of forty-seven years. Out of every one thousand babies, one hundred didn't make it to age one. In contrast, children born today will average seventy-five years of life, and only ten out of every one thousand will die before their first birthday. These findings strongly suggest that things aren't all that bad on the health front.

Deaths from influenza, pneumonia, tuberculosis, and intestinal disease have decreased dramatically. Cardiovascular diseases, including heart disease and stroke, while still accounting for a majority of deaths, have steadily declined for the past twenty-five years, a drop that started long before the recent emphasis on heart-health diets and aerobic exercise. And what about cancer?

Cancers can be divided roughly into three groups. The largest group—including cancer of the breast, colon, ovary, pancreas, bladder, and esophagus, as well as leukemia—has remained relatively unchanged in incidence for a number of years. A second group of cancers, including stomach and uterine cancer, has shown a dramatic decline. (Ironically, given today's emphasis on natural foods, there is growing speculation that the striking drop in stomach cancer may be tied to the use of anti-oxidant food preservatives such as BHT and BHA.)

The third group includes cancers showing a significant increase. There are only three: melanoma, a skin cancer related to sun exposure; prostate cancer, which is associated with an aging population; and lung cancer, caused by cigarette smoking. Of these three cancers, only lung cancer is a major killer. It has shown a steep rise over the past five decades, especially in women.

But the increase in these three cancers does not alter the overall picture. Most types of cancer have either been on the decline or remained relatively constant for the past fifty years. Dire predictions of a galloping escalation in cancer rates due to environmental pollutants have proven unfounded. Despite our deep-seated fears, there is no cancer epidemic.

So paradoxically at a time when we are living longer and enjoying healthier lives, dark images of menacing health threats come at us from all directions. Good health would seem to have little chance. What's going on? The chief culprit behind this distorted picture is health hype.

Health Hype

What is it? Health hype is like any other kind of hype. It exaggerates. It overstates the case. Whatever the facts may be, health hype feels compelled to magnify them. Minor risks become major threats. Unproven speculations about disease prevention are transformed into unequivocal prescriptions for health. Health hype doesn't understand the word subtle. Sticking to the facts is definitely less important than how the story is told. What sells determines what is newsworthy.

Health hype has made health hot. As consumers, we can't seem to get enough of it, especially health tips: quick-and-easy ways to lose weight, throw off stress, get fit, and live longer. In its commitment to entertain us, health hype feels no obligation to keep things in perspective. It ignores distinctions between the serious and the trivial. It feels no compunction about lumping together low fiber, saccharin, tampons, sugar, and smoking as equal partners in health crimes. While exotic health risks are lavishly presented, more commonplace health hazards (the ones most likely to take our lives early) are underplayed. Why? Because they are not new or dramatic. The entertainment value is gone.

Take cigarette smoking, for instance. There is no pizzazz in the dangers of cigarette smoking. They are old hat. Health hype knows very well that when it comes to what plays best, dramatic trivia is better than dull substance anytime. In its insatiable appetite for hot items, the media has difficulty handling straight health news. Increasingly, the facts about health and disease are difficult to get. But health hype is not a media exclusive. It's brought to us by an ensemble cast, each player making an essential contribution, one playing off the other.

Medical scientists have a leading role. Through the magic of statistical games, they are able and willing to meet health hype's demands for sweeping generalizations. Statistical results become tips for everyone on how to stay well. Researchers have fallen into breaching their own rules of evidence, deriving broad dictums from the results of limited studies. Most of us would like to think of medical scientists as reliable sources of important health information. Unfortunately, as we shall see, often this is not the case. The results of medical studies, even the best ones, are generalizations. With respect to individual health matters, these studies often mislead more than they inform. We will take a closer look at this problem in the next chapter when we consider the consequences of salt, cholesterol, and exercise.

But it's not just medical researchers—medical practitioners also contribute to health hype. They push the treatments and procedures that happen to be in vogue. They overtreat and over-test. The practice of medicine, among other things, is a way of making a living. As things get tight, physicians are prone to oversell their patients on questionable practices such as annual physical examinations, elaborate medical testing, extra office visits, and unnecessary surgeries. Health hype is not confined to radio, television, and the printed page.

Health hype has also worked its way on our legal and regulatory minds. Consider the Delaney Clause—the law banning the human consumption of any food substance known to cause cancer in laboratory animals (even when it requires astronomical amounts). Passed in 1958 and still operative today (despite many attempts to change it), the Delaney Clause assumes that no matter how farfetched, any risk is a significant risk from which all Americans must be protected. It's one of health hype's favorite assumptions. It was this law that banned (temporarily) saccharin from the nation's grocery-store shelves because researchers had found that a person consuming two to three cans of saccharin-sweetened soda every day of his or her life would have an increased chance of less than one in a million of getting bladder cancer! After a massive public outcry, Congress was forced to pass a special law allowing a moratorium on the saccharin ban. (The National Cancer Institute reported in 1989 in the *New York Times* that *no* cancer had been reported in laboratory monkeys, each of whom had been fed five days a week for seventeen years the amount of cyclamate contained in thirty cans of diet soda!) This is legislative health hype in action.

The courtroom has also bowed to health exaggerations. Several years ago Dan White, the killer of San Francisco mayor George Moscone and city supervisor Harvey Milk, was tried and found to suffer from diminished capacity attributable in part—so his lawyers claimed and so a psychiatrist testified—to junk food addiction. Twinkies (at least in part) made him do it.

Business is another member of the cast. There is money in health—lots of money. That's why business has been quick to jump on the bandwagon. The fitness business, with all its designer equipment and chic dresswear, has become a commercial blockbuster. On the food front, there have been many advertising coups driven by the return-to-nature idea. Natural is in. If you label something natural you can almost bank on it. Foods that have been attacked by health hype appear to have decided that "if you can't beat them, join them." Food producers have turned to natural as a survival tactic. The Sugar Association stresses that sugar is nature's official sweetener. The ads ask, "Which would you rather put on your kids' cereal?" Sugar, they point out, appears on the FDA's safe list, a claim artificial sweeteners can't make. The beef industry also tried a new slant. Their ads sported a glamorous picture of actress Cybill Shepherd, who is quoted as saying: "Sometimes I wonder if people have a primal, instinctive craving for hamburgers. Something hot and juicy and so utterly simple you can eat it with your hands."

Natural has been one of health hype's favorite lines. Later we will consider the limits of natural's claim to health.

Ironically, the other major contributors to health hype are consumers. If you want to see our eyes light up, promise us healthier and longer lives, and make the solution simple, like taking vitamins. We'll go for it every time, generation after generation, even when the promise is based on the slimmest of evidence. Robert J. Samuelson, writing for *Newsweek,* characterized it this way: "We Americans are great optimists. No one has yet devised a preventive for death, but we keep looking." As consumers we love the quick fix, the one-two-three steps to perfect health, happiness, and long life.

Consider the book *Fit for Life,* written by a man (and his wife) with a "doctorate" in "nutritional science" allegedly from an unaccredited correspondence school. After its publication in 1985, this book quickly became one of the fastest-selling diet books in history. The book's appeal is obvious: it's simple. According to the *Fit for Life* theory, fruits and vegetables should be 70 percent of the diet. Why? Because, according to the authors, they're 70 percent water, just like the human body. Furthermore, they insist only fresh fruit and juices should be eaten before noon each day to avoid overburdening the body. If you stick to this rule, you can eat as much fruit as you want. "Fruit," they say, "is the most important food that you can possibly eat!" You just have to remember never to combine it with anything else. In a nutshell, this is the "fit for life" dietary plan. So, what's the problem?

Nutritional authorities say there is not a shred of evidence to support these contentions. As ideas, they are simple, clear, and dead wrong! Nevertheless, the book's sales have been tremendous, and the sequel has already appeared. Consumers are titillated by health hype; we prefer it to the comparatively dull and often ambiguous facts about health.

Health hype has succeeded in medicalizing routine matters of living. Eating for fun and camaraderie has become passé. Calories have to be counted and food groups balanced. Taste and pleasure may have to be sacrificed. As health hype tells it, eating is serious health-promoting business.

The same with exercise. The everyday activities of living have been eclipsed by designer aerobics. If your heart doesn't go fast enough or if you don't exercise three times a week for at least twenty minutes, it doesn't count. It's inferior exercise. Whether we enjoy it or not is beside the point.

I've written this book as much for myself as anyone else. Despite my medical background, increasingly I have had difficulty making sense out of all the health warnings and panaceas. I have been hard-pressed to know how concerned to be about the newest health hazard headline; and I have long since realized there is no way I can pay attention to all health-improvement prescriptions. To do so would be to make a full-time commitment to taking care of my health. Even then I'm not certain there would be enough time or money to get the job done.

In the remaining chapters, we will take a more detailed look at how health fiction substitutes for health facts. As we do, it's important to keep this one thought in mind: Health is a highly individual matter. What's good for one person is not always good for another. And the other side is equally true. What poses a serious health risk for one person may be of little consequence to another. It depends on a lot of things. There is a strong tendency to ignore this fact, even among medical researchers who in any other setting would be quick to caution against overgeneralizing but who often fall into making sweeping pronouncements when they are telling the world about their particular research findings.

It's important to learn how to evaluate medical evidence and apply it specifically to yourself rather than trying to incorporate every health do and don't that comes along. Your health is far too important for you to pay attention to everything you are told, even by so-called experts. Many of today's most popular health tenets, when closely examined, turn out to be true only for very few of us. To pursue certain health practices or to spend a lot of effort avoiding certain risks is, at best, a waste of time and, at worse, a health hazard in its own right.

Points to Remember

1. Health hype pushes gloom and doom. Health threats make good headlines, but don't let yourself be taken in. The health of Americans is not too shabby. We are living longer and healthier lives than ever before.

2. Health hype loves simplistic answers: Take some vitamins and live an extra fifty years! There is a lot we don't know about health matters. Medical science does not have all the answers (even though it won't always admit it). It is better to accept the ambiguous state of things and use your best judgment than to let health hype do its number on you.

3. Contrary to the *Fit for Life* thesis, there is no bad food. It's all in how much you eat and how you coordinate and balance it with other foods and exercise.

4. When someone proclaims a universal health tip—good for everyone—get ready to walk away. Health is a highly individual matter. That is why getting the truth about health and disease is so difficult.

▸ ▸ ▸ ▸ ▸

Doug loathed jogging and did it because of the articles,
all that evidence about cardiovascular benefits that
would keep you alive longer. Nobody gave you an
actual number, though. Will one thousand miles of
tedious jogging give you an extra six days, six weeks?
And when do you get your jogger's bonus, he won-
dered. Now, when you're still able to eat a pastrami
sandwich, or at the end when you're already on a life-
support system?

—Avery Corman, 50

▸ ▸ ▸ ▸ ▸ ▸ ▸ ▸

CHAPTER TWO

Health Hype Hall of Fame

If there really were a Health Hype Hall of Fame, there would be no scarcity of deserving nominees. Of the many, I have selected three for special consideration.

Second runner-up goes to the smear campaign directed at salt as the cause of hypertension. Exercise as the key to long life takes the first runner-up spot; and—drum roll, please—the winner, the first inductee into the Health Hype Hall of Fame, is a remarkably flawed study that became a health news sensation as "proof" that low-cholesterol diets prevent heart disease.

The Knave of Hearts

In January of 1984, after twelve years and $150 million, what was billed as the "final" word on cholesterol and heart disease was presented in an auditorium at the National Institutes of Health filled with reporters, tape recorders, and cameras. Dr. Robert L. Levy, the man most responsible for this "watershed" research project, came right to the point. "There can no longer be any doubt," he said, "that cholesterol causes heart disease." This unequivocal conclusion echoed through the media like an orchestrated chant:

LOWERED CHOLESTEROL DECREASES HEART DISEASE
The findings are expected to affect profoundly the practices of medicine in this country.
—*Science*

HOW TO REDUCE YOUR RISK OF HEART DISEASE
[The study] demonstrated conclusively that lowering cholesterol levels helps to prevent heart attacks.
—Jane Brody, *The New York Times*

CHOLESTEROL: THE VILLAIN REVEALED
For the first time, there was direct overwhelming evidence that reducing cholesterol levels prevents heart attacks.

—Discover

THE CHOLESTEROL CONTROVERSY IS OVER
Perhaps the great epidemic of the 20th century, coronary heart disease, is about to recede.

—Dr. Peter Wood, *Runner's World*

HOLD THE EGGS AND BUTTER
Cholesterol is proved deadly.

—Claudia Wallis, *Time*

The director of the famous Framingham study of heart disease, Dr. William Castelli, had this to say when quoted in *Science Digest* (April 1985): "I think this study is going to be the breakthrough of this decade. Using the best science we can generate in medicine, this study has shown beyond a shadow of a doubt that for every one percent you lower your blood cholesterol, you lower your chances of having a heart attack by two percent."

Powerful praise and rave reviews, but, as you may have already guessed, not quite the whole story. The cholesterol study was a badly flawed piece of research that rode to international prominence on a horse named Hype.

Despite a prestigious sponsor (the National Heart, Lung, and Blood Institute), the best of intentions, and considerable time and money, the Coronary Primary Prevention Trial did not prove that cholesterol causes heart disease. Furthermore, even though the researchers claimed to have proven that all Americans should be on low-cholesterol diets, the fact is that they did not even study—much less prove—the effects of dietary cholesterol reduction. (Given the glowing reviews by the media, this may come as somewhat of a surprise!) Instead, as we shall see, the study concerned itself with a drug called cholestyramine. Somewhere along the way, this research attempt to prove the evils of eating cholesterol got sidetracked and became a drug study, a fact that the media, for the most part, still does not understand. There is indeed a difference, and it is far more than a matter of scientific hairsplitting.

As originally conceived, the study was straightforward. Several thousand middle-aged men, all with extremely high serum cholesterol levels and without any evidence as yet of heart disease, were to be divided into two comparable groups. One group then would be placed on a low-cholesterol diet and the other on a regular diet. After a lengthy interval, seven to ten years, the researchers would note any differences in the rate of heart disease and overall mortality. A good idea that never quite materialized.

At the last moment, the researchers changed their minds, most likely for two reasons. First of all, getting people to stick to a low-cholesterol diet, or any diet for that matter, for a period of years is difficult if not impossible. Second, even if such a diet is rigidly adhered to, at best it can be expected to produce only a modest reduction in serum cholesterol: on the order of 10 percent. With these reservations in mind, the researchers replaced the low-cholesterol diet with cholestyramine, a drug that predictably lowers serum cholesterol.

In short, this is how research originally slated to examine the relationship between dietary cholesterol and heart disease ended up looking at the effects of a drug. So what were the results of this widely acclaimed diet-turned-drug study?

Cholestyramine, as expected, did reduce serum cholesterol levels. So far, so good. But the true measures of the study were the comparative differences in actual heart disease and mortality. If by lowering cholesterol levels, neither was reduced, the study would hardly be considered a roaring success. Here's what was found.

In the treated group, 8.1 percent of the men came down with heart disease as compared to 9.8 percent of the controls, a difference of 1.7 percent over a period of seven to ten years. (There were twelve fewer deaths due to heart attack.) And if this result was not unimpressive enough, a comparison of the overall death rates leaves no question as to the truly undramatic nature of what this study actually showed, for the mortality rate within the two groups came within a whisker of being identical, differing only by *one-tenth of 1 percent*.

That's it: These are the "conclusive" results that supposedly established once and for all the causative role of cholesterol in heart disease and gave rise to recommendations that all men, women, and children adopt low-cholesterol diets. In actual fact, leaving out the health hype, these findings are considerably more modest in the implications.

If you are a middle-aged man with an extremely high cholesterol level and you are willing to take an expensive ($150/month), awful-tasting drug—described by one study participant as "orange-flavored sand"—six times a day for many years, you stand to lessen your chances of heart disease by 1.7 percent. (Several years later in a follow-up, it was found that three-fourths of all the men in this study had stopped taking the medication. It was that unpleasant!) And this slim advantage of 1.7 percent with respect to heart disease is offset by an increased death rate from other causes, a point somewhat glossed over by the researchers and hardly noted by the media. Paul Meier, a statistician at the University of Chicago, succinctly summed up the matter: "It was a very good study. It just had weak findings." And at Rockefeller University, Edward Ahrens, a veteran cholesterol scientist, commented: "Since this was basically a drug study, we can conclude nothing about diet; such extrapolation is unwarranted, unscientific and wishful thinking."

Matters were further clouded when it surfaced that somewhere between this study's inception and final reporting, the statistical criteria were changed! The standard was lowered. If the original standard had been adhered to, the results would not have been statistically significant, and the report likely would have never made its way into the scientific literature. As it was, it appeared courtesy of the *Journal of the American Medical Association*.

Despite these glaring deficiencies, this cholesterol story would not be denied. The cholesterol researchers pressed their case. They boldly conjectured that an estimated thirty-five to fifty million men and women could reduce their chances of heart disease by going on a low-cholesterol diet. Dr. Robert Levy, quoted in *Time*, commented: "If we can get everyone to lower his cholesterol 10 percent to 15 percent by cutting down on fat and cholesterol in the diet, heart attack deaths in this country will decrease by 20 percent to 30 percent." Why the good doctor felt he could speak for everyone based on a study of men with very high cholesterol levels is not readily apparent. He and others, including the American Heart Association, have used this study to recommend that all children over the age of two go on low-cholesterol diets. To give them the benefit of the doubt, perhaps these authorities are going beyond this particular study and relying on other research. Unfortunately, here too they are on somewhat shaky ground.

In a January 1985 article entitled "Heart Panel's Conclusions Questioned," Gina Kolata, a reporter for *Science,* pointed out that over the past twenty years, close to two dozen major clinical trials of cholesterol reduction had been conducted. These studies have involved more than fifty thousand people at high risk for heart disease—the very people most likely to show benefit if there is benefit to be had. But they, like the Coronary Primary Prevention Trial, have failed to show that lowering cholesterol substantially reduces deaths from heart disease. Moreover, even if you throw all these studies together and look for an overall positive effect, you still cannot see one. The small reduction in mortality from coronary heart disease is fully offset by an increase in deaths from noncoronary diseases such as colon cancer.

More recently Harvard researchers, reporting in *Annals of Internal Medicine,* have projected the increase in life expectancy that could result from cholesterol reduction. They prefaced their results with the caveat that their study assumed that cholesterol reduction is effective and safe. Perhaps these assumptions are correct, perhaps they are not; either way, the results were meager. After a lifelong program of cholesterol reduction, persons aged twenty to sixty years who were low risk for heart disease could expect to live an extra three days to three months. For individuals at high risk, the gain ranged from eighteen days to twelve months.

Despite claims to the contrary, the great cholesterol study wasn't what it was cracked up to be. The real story was not that "the cholesterol controversy is over," but rather that the National Institutes of Health spent a fortune on a flawed study that proved *nothing* about dietary cholesterol and heart disease, and still managed to sweep the media off its feet. To this day this study is widely quoted in both the scientific and popular media as proof that a low-cholesterol diet reduces heart disease. In 1985, based on the study's "findings," the federal government launched a massive educational campaign known as the National Cholesterol Education Program aimed at getting all American adults to adopt a low-cholesterol diet.

All in all, an impressive piece of health fiction. And I would not count on ever seeing a correction notice such as "Conclusions from Landmark Cholesterol Study in Error." Millions of taxpayers' dollars were spent, research careers made, and astronomical commercial profits realized as a result of the unwarranted conclusions drawn from this study. So the first inductee into the Health Hype Hall of Fame likely will remain the study that "proved" low-cholesterol diets are the key to preventing heart disease.

No Pain, No Gain

First runner-up for the Health Hype Hall of Fame is a popular maxim now engraved in stone as health truth: "Exercise to live longer."

Aerobic exercise has taken the country by storm. Health clubs multiply like rabbits, and month after month new books and video-tapes championing various exercise routines appear as best-sellers. A host of media celebrities have made new careers in the exercise business. Marathons have become contemporary "happenings," and jogging paraphernalia has emerged as a billion-dollar business.

Millions of Americans are vigorously exercising, many of them with visions of life extension dancing in their heads. While there's little doubt that regular exercise has some important benefits, longer life, as it turns out, is probably *not* one of them.

Henry A. Solomon, a practicing cardiologist on the faculty of Cornell University Medical College, has written a highly readable book on the overselling of exercise entitled *The Exercise Myth*. I won't keep you in suspense, but will go right to the punch line: "It [exercise] will not make you live longer." But if Dr. Solomon is right, how did the idea of a link between exercise and long life get started? It's an intriguing story.

According to Dr. Solomon, the first major report on the health benefits of exercise dates back to 1953. Jeremy Morris at the London Hospital co-authored a paper in the British medical journal *Lancet* entitled "Coronary Heart Disease and Physical Activity of Work." Morris and his colleagues devised a simple way of looking at the health benefits of exercise. They convinced themselves that London transit workers afforded them a perfect natural experiment. This was their reasoning: London bus drivers, glued to their seats all day as they were, led a far more sedentary life than their counterparts, the conductors, who, as part of their jobs, were constantly jumping on and off the bus, collecting fares, and telling people where the bus was going and where to get off—all the time moving between the first and second levels of the world-famous double-decker London buses.

In all, thirty-one thousand drivers and conductors had their subsequent rates of heart disease compared. At the conclusion the researchers found that their conjecture had been correct: drivers suffered considerably *more* heart disease than conductors. From this result it was concluded that physical activity did indeed provide protection from heart disease. Oddly enough, at the time this conclusion did not get much public attention (my, how things have changed), but it did not go unnoticed by health professionals. It is still described in textbooks as a classic study.

What did not gain much subsequent attention, as is so often the case, was a second report from Morris and his colleagues three years later in *Lancet* which greatly qualified his original conclusions. Why? Because he and his colleagues had discovered that the drivers were physiologically different from conductors at the outset of the study. They had more risk factors for heart disease *before* their years of London transit work and therefore would have been expected to show higher rates of heart disease, regardless of the amount of physical activity. Morris, by his own admission, had studied a biased sample, the bane of all researchers, thus bringing into serious question his original conclusion. But the qualification made little difference. The idea that physical activity was the road to longer life was on the books. It wouldn't go away. (There is an important lesson here. Initial "medical breakthroughs" have a way of getting headlines; retractions don't fare nearly as well. As with the cholesterol study, years often pass without corrections being made of erroneous research findings.)

Other investigations gave further impetus to the idea that exercise lengthens one's life. In the early sixties, at the University of Minnesota, H. L. Taylor and others examined the records of railroad workers and found lower death rates in the most active men. Similarly, a study from the Health Insurance Plan of Greater New York found that twice as many sedentary men could expect to have a first heart attack compared to those who participated in at least moderate exercise.

In the seventies, Dr. Thomas J. Bassler, a California pathologist and devoted marathoner, became so taken with the heart-health benefits of long-distance running he proposed the "marathon hypothesis." According to Bassler, if you clocked in enough miles of running, you could be sure you wouldn't die from coronary heart disease. The marathon hypothesis, although never substantiated, hung around until the 1984 death of Jim Fixx, author of *The Complete Book of Running*. Fixx, a devoted long-distance runner, collapsed and died immediately of a heart attack while jogging in northern Vermont. On autopsy, he was found to have severe arteriosclerotic heart disease, a condition prevalent in his family and one from which, as it was later revealed, he had been suffering symptoms for some time. Heart attacks and early cardiac deaths do occur in athletes, reminding us that fitness, contrary to the marathon hypothesis, does not provide absolute immunity against coronary heart disease.

Investigations into the health benefits of exercise have produced mixed results. In contrast to some positive reports, several major studies have not only failed to find in favor of exercise, they have also turned up evidence that exercise, particularly if it is heavy, actually shortens life. A 1957 study of 2,252 Los Angeles public employees found 30 percent *fewer* new cases of coronary heart disease in sedentary workers and 38 percent *more* cases than expected among men most vigorously engaged in physical activity.

Countering the earlier study of railroad workers, a 1967 analysis of Indian railway workers, appearing in the *British Heart Journal*, showed an "unexpected and extraordinary finding . . . that mortality in the sedentary occupation of clerks is lower than the physically active occupation of fitters. . . . this is contrary to the current conceptions of the protective role of exercise."

More recently, the popular press picked up a *New England Journal of Medicine* report on the exercise habits of almost 1,700 Harvard alumni. *Newsweek* headlined it "Running for Your Life: A Harvard Study Links Exercise with Longevity." *Time* was even more exuberant, declaring "Extra Years for Extra Effort: A New Study Shows that Exercise Can Indeed Increase Longevity." None of the headlines mentioned the obvious: men destined to live the longest would likely be more physically robust and therefore more active. Increased exercise may have been the result of greater physical robustness rather than the cause. Given the design of the study, it's impossible to know which is which. But the headlines decided to go with the exercise-gives-extra-life idea.

Another important point was underplayed, pertaining to the actual number of years gained (presumably) due to extra exercise. Based on this study, if a physically active man survived to age eighty, he would have lived *one or two more years* than he would have had he led a sedentary life. Granted, a couple of extra years are not to be dismissed lightly; but, as one commentator wryly observed, the extra years of life you would derive are just about equal to the time you would spend exercising. In other words, it's a "wash."

Medical research studies are not infallible. Typically, contradictory findings exist side by side. This is the rule, not the exception. That's why, despite what health hype would have us believe, no single study can be trusted. The best we can do is to watch for trends. When taken together, what do the studies seem to say? Is there a preponderance of evidence one way or the other, or is the picture consistently clouded by contradiction? With respect to exercise and its effect on how long a person lives, medical researchers have failed to produce compelling evidence one way or the other. Taken together, the findings cancel out.

This is not so dissimilar from the status of cholesterol research. No matter how much we would like definitive answers to questions about exercise and long life and dietary cholesterol and heart disease, there are none. Health hype, knowing that ambiguity seldom sits well with most of us, takes each new study as it is made public and treats what it says as the whole truth. But medical truths don't pop up every day; they emerge slowly. Better to accept the ambiguity than to act as though a single study tells the whole story.

That a case for the life-extending benefits of exercise has not been made does not negate the other worthwhile benefits that can be derived from exercise. Personally, I don't let the lack of evidence stop me from jogging regularly. I do it because it makes me feel good, keeps me physically fit, and helps control my weight. These benefits are more than enough to keep me exercising. The promise of longer life I simply file away in my folder marked "Health Hype." Possible, but not proven.

Later we will consider the hidden health risks that many "tips for health" carry with them. Exercise (particularly certain kinds) is no exception. It's important to keep these invisible costs in mind when considering the overall health value of anything.

Salt: The Table Poison

Second runner-up for the Health Hype Hall of Fame is that smear campaign that's been methodically carried out against salt. In a relatively short time, table salt has gone from being considered a harmless flavor enhancer to being labeled health poison. Book stores are filled with diatribes against salt: *Killer Salt; Halt! No Salt; Shake the Salt Habit; Salt: The Demon Crystal*. Salt-as-poison has become a major plank in our health platform and has launched a booming business in low-salt foods.

A link between salt and hypertension has been suspected for more than eighty years. Much of the evidence, however, is indirect. For example, studies have shown that in some countries where food is highly salted, high blood pressure is more prevalent than in countries with low salt intake. The Japanese, for example, with their sizable consumption of fish, pickled vegetables, and soy sauce, consume lots of salt; and high blood pressure, along with one of its sequelae, stroke, is quite prevalent in Japan. Conversely, populations such as the Yanomamo Indians of Brazil, who eat virtually no salt, have almost no cases of high blood pressure. (I would add, however, that other population studies have found the opposite results. Buddhist farmers in Thailand who consume large quantities of rice with a high salt intake maintain normal blood pressures into old age. Also, sugar-plantation workers of St. Kitts, despite drinking only stored rainwater and having less than half the salt intake of Buddhist rice farmers, commonly suffer from high blood pressure.)

But there's a problem with all of these studies. Their findings are only statistical. More than likely, other things besides salt consumption distinguish the Yanomamo Indians from the Japanese and other people with high blood pressure. The link between salt intake and high blood pressure could well be a misleading correlation, masking the true causative culprit.

One thing seems certain, salt affects different people in different ways. It is now widely recognized that certain individuals who already suffer from high blood pressure will have a worsening of their condition if they consume extra salt. Similarly, these same individuals may find that their blood pressure drops if they have less salt. But this is not true of all persons with high blood pressure, only of a fraction. Of the roughly one out of five American adults who have high blood pressure, only about half are "salt-sensitive"; that is, their blood pressure reacts adversely to salt and can be lowered by consuming less of it.

What about the rest of us, who either do not have high blood pressure or have a form that is not salt-sensitive? For the vast majority of us—close to 90 percent—salt is simply not a problem, despite the media's insistence that salt is poison.

High blood pressure is not well understood. It is clear, however, that it does not arise from a single cause. High blood pressure is a syndrome resulting from a number of different causes including genetic predisposition. It's not clear that salt ever *causes* high blood pressure, but if it does, it is only in certain persons, most likely related to their genetics, according to an article in the *American Journal of Clinical Nutrition*. For most of us, salt is harmless; we are not going to develop high blood pressure, period, regardless of how many salty snacks we eat. Our bodies will handle it. After all, salt is about as common a substance as you can find. Fully 70 percent of our body weight is salt water.

How difficult is it to give a normal person high blood pressure by feeding him or her loads of salt? Very difficult. One study, reported in *Science*, gave healthy men seventy-five grams of salt a day, an amount fifteen times greater than the average daily consumption. Even so, the men did not develop high blood pressure. What happened to all the salt? Their bodies, largely through the work of their kidneys, simply got rid of the extra salt by excreting larger amounts into the urine. In those few cases where slight rises in blood pressure occurred, it quickly returned to normal when potassium was added and stayed down even when the salt loading was continued.

Most of us can, and do, eat lots of salt without negative health consequences. Which brings me to the question raised by Dr. Harriet Dustan, past president of the American Heart Association, in the same *Science* article: "Why in the name of heaven should we restrict sodium intake of people who are not hypertensive?" It's not that there is anything to be gained by eating loads of salt—I'm not suggesting that. The point is there is no need for the vast majority of us to obsess about whether or not to use the salt shaker when we want to. For most of us, salt restriction has no great health benefit.

Beating up on salt has become a favorite national pastime because it is convenient. It implies that there is a simple solution to what is actually a highly complex and poorly understood medical problem. Eat too much salt, get high blood pressure; avoid salt, avoid high blood pressure. It has a certain ring to it. It makes a medical condition afflicting millions of Americans easy to understand, easy to write about, and easy to prescribe for. Unfortunately, it's not a correct explanation.

Also, salt restriction has become big business. The selling of low-salt foods and salt substitutes is highly profitable. Advertising bases its appeal on the alleged health benefits of low salt. Consider the consequences if tomorrow the nonrelationship between salt and high blood pressure were clarified, emphasizing that salt-sensitive persons are small in number and that for the rest of us, salt is not a health hazard. Profits of a host of companies would be jeopardized, a turn of events stockholders would not find amusing. Salt researchers would have some sleepless nights, and millions of consumers who have come to feel comfortable in their avoidance of the salt shaker would experience a sense of betrayal. (It's easy to see how once health hype takes hold, it resists change with a vengeance. There's a lot riding on it.)

In the summer of 1984, the journal *Science* carried a report, "Blood Pressure and Nutrient Intake in the United States," by Dr. David McCarron, director of the Hypertension Program at Oregon Health Sciences University, and his colleagues. These researchers performed a computer analysis of the relationship of seventeen nutrients to blood pressure. Their subjects were 10,372 adults, aged eighteen to seventy-four, who denied any history of hypertension or the use of special diets. Based on self-reports of what they had eaten over a twenty-four-hour period, plus a medical examination, an intriguing and unexpected profile emerged.

One out of every ten of these subjects turned out to have high blood pressure. But instead of being associated with excessive dietary sodium, the opposite was true. High blood pressure was lowest among persons consuming the most salt and other sodium-containing foods and highest among those consuming low amounts of sodium.

The most surprising finding, however, had nothing to do with sodium: it concerned calcium. "Lower calcium intake was the most consistent factor in hypertensive individuals. Across the population, higher intakes of calcium, potassium, and sodium were associated with lower mean systolic blood pressure and lower absolute risk of hypertension."

Despite Dr. McCarron's care in emphasizing that his results did not prove that low dietary calcium causes high blood pressure, the study drew quick fire from government officials, food companies, and consumer groups. Questions about the validity of dietary recall were raised. Officials pointed out how this study "flew in the face of" most previous studies. The attacks grew even nastier when it was discovered that Dr. McCarron receives a small amount of his funding (6 percent) from the dairy industry (pro-calcium!).

If it turns out that low calcium is tied to high blood pressure, then the advice many Americans have been given about avoiding high-salt, high-sodium foods may well have been counterproductive. That's because many calcium-rich foods (such as baked goods) are high in sodium. As these foods were avoided in order to keep sodium and salt intake down, calcium was also reduced.

But as I've cautioned, no single study tells the truth of things, and McCarron's study is no exception. Alone it cannot make the case against salt's role in high blood pressure. But it reminds us of an important point: the facts are not all in on salt and high blood pressure.

Like the majority of Americans, I don't have high blood pressure and it doesn't run in my family. So I salt food to suit my taste. If I should ever develop high blood pressure, it would be reasonable (at least on a trial basis) to see if salt restriction would help. Until that time, I don't see any reason to get too worked up over how much salt I'm eating each day.

Points to Remember

1. Many of our most cherished health beliefs rest more on the shoulders of health hype than on solid scientific evidence.

2. Of the host of excellent candidates for the Health Hype Hall of Fame, my top three are: cholesterol as the "knave of

hearts"; exercise as the key to long life; and salt as the cause of high blood pressure. There are plenty more.

3. The best of medical studies are vulnerable to hype, and some of the best researchers are not above participating in it. It's good for the career. So, in the tradition of "trust everyone but tie your camel to the tree," question everything.

4. No matter how prestigious the sponsor or the researchers involved, single studies are extremely limited in what they can tell us. Medical truths are slow in coming, and even when they arrive they are tentative.

5. Overgeneralization is rampant. (We will return to this theme in chapter 7, which discusses statistical games.)

6. Medical research retractions seldom appear, and when they do, they usually don't make the front page.

▶ ▶ ▶ ▶ ▶

It worries me greatly, but the facts don't seem to help much. People just have an inappropriate sense of what is dangerous. They get overly upset about minor problems. If you translate the weight and time it takes a laboratory rat to develop bladder cancer to a 200-pound man drinking Fresca, it comes out to about two bathtubs full each day. People dropped Fresca in a minute, but they continue to smoke.

—Surgeon General C. Everett Koop,
quoted in *Los Angeles Times,*
May 9, 1989

CHAPTER THREE

▸ ▸ ▸ ▸ ▸ ▸ ▸ ▸ ▸

The Health-Risk Jungle

Don't let all the health risks in the headlines scare you. Most of them are full of generalizations and ambiguities—in fact, the worry they cause you is probably more dangerous than the "risks" themselves. This chapter gives you guidelines that will help you distinguish real concerns from trivia.

The first guideline is this: *Accept the fact that some risk is a part of everyday living.* Whether you're driving to work, working in the garden, or shoveling snow, you are at some risk of becoming injured or dying. Even "safe" activities like singing in the shower, washing the dishes, and sleeping in bed, pose some risk of injury. Unless a new health hazard is riskier than these day-to-day risks of ordinary living, it should not be given more than passing interest, no matter who is crying "wolf." And even then, the evidence should be compelling, which usually means more than a single medical study.

Remember: keep your perspective. Ask yourself, what are the *actual* odds of it affecting you? And even if your risk is ten times greater than someone else's, if the chances of its happening to you are still minuscule, it's not worth losing sleep over.

The Answers Aren't All In

Let's move on to a second guideline: *Develop a tolerance for ambiguity.* Health and disease are complicated matters. Despite the wonders of high-tech medical research and the promises of holistic medicine, much remains unknown. It would not be so bad if all the players were willing to own up to this fact, but that's not the case. Ask any question about how to stay well and live a long life, and I guarantee someone will step forward to give you a "definitive" answer. In the health field, far more is claimed with unswerving confidence than the evidence merits.

And I am not just speaking of the "health evangelists." The lack of sound answers applies equally well to the experts. This is not to put down the contributions of medical research. Many of them are truly awesome; nevertheless, there are serious limits to how medical science can reasonably advise individuals. Many research findings are based on averages that are difficult, if not impossible, to apply individually. It is these averages that, more often than not, become headlines. While the implication is that we all should take heed, the truth is that these findings typically have relevance only for a very few individuals.

When we don't have answers (particularly about something as important as our health), it is tempting to just accept whatever comes along. Someone tells us everything will be okay; if we just take a load of vitamins, we'll be 100 percent better. No one is giving us any better answers, and, after all, it's only vitamins. Rather than resist, it's easier to make the purchase. But for most health "prescriptions"—even vitamins—there are hidden risks, sometimes serious ones. The admonitions of health fiction can themselves be hazardous to our health.

In the midst of the health-risk jungle, we are far better off putting the burden of evidence on whoever is doing the selling. If they cannot make the case on something more than strong conviction, it's best to say, "No, thank you," and move on—even if that means going without an answer for a while longer. When we cannot tolerate ambiguity, health hype has a field day.

Don't Trust the Headlines

A third guideline relates to bias we have in approaching health risks: *Don't let the flair for drama overly influence you.* This is a difficult guideline because, like the media, we are overly sensitive to dramatic health hazards and relatively insensitive to more mundane threats, even when the latter merit far more concern.

The major killer diseases, almost by definition, are commonplace. They don't get their share of headlines; they just quietly kill us by the thousands. Alcohol, for example, plays a major role in cirrhosis of the liver and automobile accidents (two of the top ten causes of death) and contributes to homicide, suicide, and several kinds of cancer. Alcohol is so much a part of our social fabric we don't even think of it as a drug.

Similarly, when people are asked to give comparisons between the number of deaths from several chronic diseases and more exotic causes of death, typically the responses are quite distorted. Deaths from chronic diseases such as asthma, emphysema, and diabetes are grossly underestimated while deaths due to homicide, botulism, and tornadoes are exaggerated. The more sensational a cause of death, the more likely it is that its occurrence will be overestimated. In one study, individuals queried about homicide and stroke attributed more deaths to homicide, while in reality, ten times as many people die from strokes! The same study asked about asthma and tornadoes: how many victims of each are there annually in the United States? On the average, people judged that both tornadoes and asthma kill about five hundred people. The fact is that three thousand people die annually from asthma, six times as many as die from tornadoes.

We know from headlines that the media shares that bias for the unusual at the expense of the more common. A study of two newspapers showed that news coverage did not come close to reflecting the actual frequency of death from various causes. News space devoted to accidental death was six times greater than that given to death from heart disease and cancer even though these two diseases caused more than sixteen times as many deaths. The same principle is at work in the pages of magazines and in radio and television news. Health items are covered more for their entertainment value than for their newsworthiness. This is why if our knowledge is based on health fiction rather than fact, we run the risk of compounding our natural tendency to give spectacular health threats far more attention than they deserve.

The Dread Factor

The sensational is not the only means by which health hype seduces us. It also uses those things that seem to be beyond our control. Researchers have estimated that we will assume ten to one hundred times more risk when we perceive it to be voluntary rather than involuntary. This is probably why some of us enthusiastically take on the dangers of downhill skiing, motorcycling, or hang gliding, yet express grave concern about food preservatives, artificial sweeteners, food irradiation, and water impurities. These latter things seem imposed on us, beyond our control.

In February 1986 nearly two million Americans who had planned trips abroad suddenly changed their minds. Why? Because of a widely publicized instance of terrorism. Most of the changes in travel plans were made out of fear of being the victims of terrorism. The odds of this happening were remote; in fact, more Americans drowned in their own bathtubs the preceding year than were killed by terrorists. The risk of terrorist attack seemed greater (at least in part) because terrorism is something done to us. It is a threat beyond our control; the kind of threat we fear the most.

Analysts at Decision Research Corporation in Eugene, Oregon, call it the "Dread Factor." This is the term they have coined for this exaggerated fear of risks thought to be outside our control. They suggest that it's the dread factor that comes into play in our evaluation of health hazards like nuclear generated electrical power.

Although nuclear power raises a number of realistic concerns, some of our fears do relate to our poor understanding of it. For most of us, nuclear power is an unknown and sinister force, capable of rising up any moment in a Chernobyl-like nightmare and destroying thousands of people. But its track record (at least in this country) doesn't support our fear.

In thirty years there have been three deaths in the United States directly attributable to nuclear power plants. Contrast this to deaths connected with the more widely used power source, coal. Each year about 150 coal miners die in mining accidents alone. Many more die of coal-related lung disease. When all deaths related to coal are added together, including transportation and air pollution from coal-burning power sources, experts estimate that the cost in human life for coal-generated electricity runs over one hundred thousand people per year. The case could be made that it's the dread factor at work that tips the balance in favor of a more destructive energy source. We need to keep the dread factor in check, or we will consistently exaggerate technological dangers we do not fully understand, while tending to minimize the commonplace hazards that kill us before our time.

Because we approach health risks with strong subjective preconceptions, we are prone to glaring inconsistencies in our interpretations of various health risks. William Allman, in a *Science 85* article entitled "Staying Alive in the 20th Century," summarized it this way: "It's the same general public that smokes billions of cigarettes a year while banning an artificial sweetener because of a one-in-a-million chance that it might cause cancer; the same public that eats meals full of fat, flocks to cities prone to earthquakes, and goes hang gliding while it frets about pesticides in foods, avoids the ocean for fear of sharks, and breaks into a cold sweat on airline flights. In short, we the general public are irrational, uninformed, superstitious, even stupid. We don't understand probability, are biased by the news media, and have a fear of some technologies that borders on the primeval." Strong words.

If tomorrow a fully loaded 747 airplane should go down between Los Angeles and New York City, crashing without survivors, this tragedy would be the center of media attention for days. For the next week or so airline travel would decrease while purchases of air-travel insurance would surge.

Contrast this with the attention given to cigarette smoking, a prolonged and less dramatic catastrophe. Each year in the United States alone cigarette smoking causes roughly half a million premature deaths. In their book *Risk Watch: The Odds of Life*, authors John Urquhart and Klaus Heilmann pointed out that this is the equivalent of three fully loaded 747s crashing without survivors each day! The loss of life from commercial airplane crashes is infinitesimal compared to that from cigarette smoking. But the headlines go to air crashes. The result is that air travel takes on far more risk in our minds than is justified and cigarette smoking far too little.

Fear of flying is one of the more common phobias of our time. The facts (while generally of little help in allaying phobic concerns) provide considerable evidence for reassurance. One way of stating the risk is in terms of the increased chances of dying in a given year. For example, taking a one-thousand-mile jet flight increases a person's annual likelihood of dying by one in a million. Another approach is to look at the odds of any single passenger dying in a plane crash. Between the years 1974 and 1979, 1,468,000,000 persons traveled on commercial airliners in the United States. During that same period there were roughly 1,800 crash deaths. If we divide the number of passengers by the number of victims, we find that one out of every 814,000 passengers died in commercial plane crashes! Those are awfully good odds.

It's All in How the Facts Are Presented

We come to a fourth guideline: *When you are considering health facts, look for alternative ways of interpreting them.* Consider this example. You hear a doctor report on television the latest study showing that women on birth control pills have eight times greater risk of circulatory disease, namely heart attacks and strokes. It sounds serious. But before you stop the pill (or if you are a man, before you encourage your wife or lover to stop the pill), take another look at what's been said. Not much, really; at least, not enough to tell us how serious the risk really is.

First, we need to know how frequently circulatory diseases occur in women who *don't* take the pill. If it turns out that it's a common occurrence, then the fact that it is eight times more likely in women on the pill would be of great concern. But in actuality, this is not the case. The chances are small that a thirty-year-old woman who is not on the pill and does not smoke will develop heart disease or a stroke. How rare? Roughly 1 out of 37,000. So even though a thirty-year-old woman has eight times the risk, that still makes her chances come out to only 8 out of 37,000. Certainly not something to be overly concerned about. (We will return to this point later in chapter 7 when we discuss one of health hype's favorite tools, *relative risk.*) In fact, the risk is even less because it's mainly the older women on the pill who smoke that have circulatory problems. The figure of eight times greater risk is an overall average that grossly overstates the danger for younger, nonsmoking women. For most nonsmoking women under the age of thirty-five, using an oral contraceptive is less risky than driving an automobile. (The few exceptions would be those women who have a strong family history of circulatory disease.)

The point of all this is that health fiction hardly ever gives us all the relevant facts, and what it does tell us is often framed in such a way that risks or benefits, as the case may be, are exaggerated. If we are not to be misled by health fiction, we have to look for the rest of the story, and we have to consider different interpretations. This may mean reading other reports, checking out other commentators, or seeking out second medical opinions. If you are seriously considering taking action on the basis of a new health report, getting additional input is definitely indicated.

Let's look at another hypothetical example. Based on his research, a medical expert claims that ten out of one hundred subjects are at risk if they don't change, let's say, their eating habits. Right off we know that an equally valid contention can be made by turning the facts around: Even if they don't change their ways, ninety out of one hundred subjects are *not* at risk. Now, this may not greatly affect your reaction to what the researcher has said, but it certainly puts things in a different perspective, which is important. More often than not, researchers won't do this for us; and even if they do, sensational reporting may ignore it. When evaluating health information, we need to get in the habit of reframing the facts ourselves, and, if possible, filling in the missing pieces. This practice alone gives us a significant advantage when trying to counter the distortions of health hype.

We are extremely susceptible to the way health information is presented. Shockingly so. This makes it even more imperative that we make a concerted effort to reframe the facts we are given. The same facts presented two slightly different ways have been shown to lead reasonable people to reverse themselves on important, albeit hypothetical, treatment decisions.

In one study described in the *New England Journal of Medicine,* 1,153 persons were asked to assume that they had been diagnosed as having lung cancer. Based on actual statistical-outcome data, they were offered two alternative treatments. A doctor explained the available treatment options: surgery or radiation. He told them that of those people who underwent surgery for lung cancer, ten out of every one hundred died during the operation, and, subsequently over the next five years, sixty-six more died. This treatment outcome was then contrasted with that obtained with radiation. While none of the radiation patients died during the treatment, over the next five years there were seventy-eight deaths. Given these statistics, the subjects were asked to select a treatment. Radiation was chosen by 44 percent.

After this choice was made, the doctor went on to present the same information in a different version, but disguised by the claim that it came from a newer study. This new information, the doctor said, confirmed the risk of dying from treatment: 10 percent in the case of surgery; 0 percent with radiation. But as for life expectancy, the newer study had found that those who survived surgery lived 6.8 years, while those who had undergone radiation survived 4.7

years. Upon hearing this second presentation, the percentage of subjects who picked radiation dropped from 44 percent to 25 percent. The subjects included radiologists, graduate students who had completed courses in statistics and decision theory, and patients at a Veterans Administration outpatient center. The framing of the facts in different ways affected both knowledgeable and unsophisticated subjects alike.

The moral to this study (and others like it) is that our decision-making skills with respect to health matters are fragile. Our best bet for ensuring sound health decisions for ourselves is to get the facts in as many different versions as we can before making up our minds.

Risk Factors Are Not All the Same

In recent years, the number of things identified as "risk factors" has mushroomed. The problem is that the term has not been adequately defined. Currently, anything that has been statistically associated with a certain disease or condition qualifies as a risk factor. If someone discovers that people who eat celery have more of a certain disease—even if it's only by a slight and inconsequential degree— celery gets catalogued as a risk factor. Thus, there are many trivial risk factors.

Even major risk factors are not well conceptualized. How many people know, for example, that many of the risk factors we hear so much about are not present in a majority of the cases of disease they have been associated with? Furthermore, in most instances it is not clear that the risk factor actually plays a causal role in the disease.

Consider the three major risk factors associated with coronary heart disease: elevated serum cholesterol, high blood pressure, and smoking. While it's true that people who have these factors are more prone to coronary heart disease, the majority of people who develop coronary heart disease do not, I repeat, *do not,* have these risk factors. So, it's highly unlikely—in fact it's impossible—that these three major heart disease risk factors actually cause heart disease. They may aggravate it, but they can hardly be considered causal when the disease commonly occurs in their absence.

Risk factors should more appropriately be thought of as markers or indicators. They identify people who are particularly susceptible to a certain disease. Although we cannot say with confidence that people without the major risk factors will not get heart disease, we can confidently predict the development of heart disease in many people who have all of them. They are eight times more susceptible to the number-one cause of death in this country.

Perhaps the following analogy will make this point more clearly: A young woman passes you on the street. She is stylishly dressed, wearing expensive jewelry, and smelling of very expensive perfume. She steps off the curb and gets into a chauffeured limousine. You surmise she is wealthy or, at least, has access to wealth. Not a bad bet. What you can't do is conclude that her expensive trappings are the "cause" of her wealth. That would be backward thinking, which is what occurs with respect to risk factors. Like the woman's rich trappings, which augment her wealth, some risk factors may actually add to the disease with which they are associated, but they are not likely the cause itself.

Health fiction doesn't see it this way. It routinely assumes that risk factors cause disease. It's a misleading assumption that may well explain why large-scale attempts to prevent diseases by treating risk factors have failed to yield convincing results.

Consider, for example, the $115,000,000, ten-year study funded by the federal government called the Multiple Risk Factor Intervention Trial, commonly known as the "MR. FIT" study. More than twelve thousand men participated. They were selected because they had all three of the major risk factors for heart disease (smoking, high blood pressure, and high cholesterol levels). Half of the men received treatment that reduced the three risk factors, compared to the other half who received nothing special. It was assumed that the treated group would have fewer deaths from heart disease over the years. It didn't turn out that way. Ten years later there was no real difference between the two groups in the number of deaths from heart disease. "MR. FIT" illustrates how risk factors often respond beautifully while the incidence of a disease continues unabated.

Recall our discussion in chapter 2 on cholesterol. There is no doubt that people who have high cholesterol levels are more prone to heart disease. That doesn't mean that the high cholesterol necessarily causes it. Perhaps the high cholesterol is merely a reflection of a more basic disturbance in the way cholesterol is handled in the body so that more cholesterol is deposited in cells than is carried away. Regardless of how high the person's serum cholesterol, given this basic defect, cholesterol will likely accumulate in places where it has no business being—like the walls of coronary arteries—and eventually will lead to the obstruction of blood flow and subsequently to a heart attack. In some individuals this may happen without the indicator of high serum cholesterol ever appearing. While this accumulation may proceed more rapidly if the cholesterol is higher, and more slowly if it is lowered, cholesterol is not the cause. (The proof is in the fact that frequently people who have heart attacks do not have high cholesterol levels.) People who don't have the fundamental defect, regardless of how much cholesterol they consume, likely will never have heart disease. Mind you, this is all speculative, but as a hypothesis it fits the facts about as well as the contention that high cholesterol causes heart disease.

So the fifth guideline is this: *Don't automatically assume that modifying a risk factor will reduce the likelihood of a disease.*

Try to Get the Bigger Picture

I will warn you at the outset, our last guideline is more easily said than done! *As much as possible, keep health risks in perspective.* Maintaining perspective is essential to making our way through the health-risk jungle; but, it is a devilish problem, in large measure, because it's so difficult to individualize risks. As I will say a number of times, health risks do not have the same consequence for everyone. One man's health risk is another man's pleasure.

There's another problem in getting a reasonable perspective. It has to do with the translation of scientifically stated risk into terms we can better grasp. Several years ago, when he was director of the Environmental Protection Agency, William Ruckelshaus commented in the journal *Science,* "We must search for ways to describe risk as clearly as possible, tell people what the known or suspected health problems are, and help them compare that risk to those with which they are more familiar."

Ruckelshaus was right on target. Straight numerical expressions of risk are severely limited in what we can make of them. Think about it: how meaningful is it to read that your risk is 1 in 6,500? Is that good or bad? Does it mean that you are highly likely to encounter the problem—unless something is done to avoid it—or does it indicate you can forget it because it's such a remote possibility? How are you supposed to feel when a medical researcher concludes that individuals who drink your favorite beverage are 158 times more likely to come down with a serious bacterial infection? It sounds bad, but exactly how risky is it? You cannot really be sure.

Consider the following: You are a forty-year-old woman, thinking about having a baby. Today's newspaper headlines in the health section announce that women your age have ten times greater chance of having a baby with Down's Syndrome. What do you make of it? Should you forget it and adopt, or go without? Or perhaps you are a parent who reads that 1 out of 310,000 children who are immunized against whooping cough (pertussis) by vaccine has a serious neurological reaction—what do you do? Is the risk great enough for you to forego having your child immunized? Does it offset the risk of your child coming down with whooping cough?

These are the kinds of health-risk questions that commonly face us. They do not always have straightforward answers, but we have to make decisions about them anyway. We need the best information we can get to put these risks into perspective.

Although the job remains unfinished, there have been some pre-liminary attempts at translating health risks into more practical terms that we can better grasp. Paul Slovic has commented on the difficulties of understanding what one part in a billion means. (Somehow 1/1,000,000,000 does not do the job.) It would be much easier to imagine, Slovic maintains, if it were stated as a one-crouton-in-a-ten-ton-salad relationship. In this spirit I have assembled in the following pages several different approaches to portraying health risks. They are a good start and point the way to more sophisticated methods (perhaps drawing on the power of computers) for putting health risks into proper perspective.

"Days Off Your Life" shows health risks in terms of the decrease in life expectancy associated with certain activities, situations, and diseases. Keep in mind that these are statistical averages and suffer from overgeneralization. They should be seen as ballpark estimates.

At the top of the list is the risk associated with being an unmarried male. On the average this state of affairs is associated with a loss of 3,500 days or almost 10 years! This top listing may come as a surprise, but there is considerable evidence that "going it alone" is risky business with respect to health. This is not to say unmarrieds are necessarily alone and isolated; but, statistically, aloneness is overrepresented among unmarrieds, both men and women. What cannot be said for certain is how much of this is cause and how much is

Table 1. Days off Your Life

	Estimated Decrease in Life Expectancy from:	
Activities and Situations	Days Lost	Diseases and Accidents
Unmarried male	3,500	
Smoking cigarettes (men)	2,250	
	2,100	Heart disease
Unmarried female	1,600	
Working as a coal miner	1,100	
	980	Cancer
20% overweight	900	
Being poor	700	
	520	Stroke
Army in Vietnam	400	
100 extra calories/day	210	
Driving a motor vehicle	207	
	141	Pneumonia, influenza
	130	Alcohol
	90	Homicide
Misusing *legal* drugs	90	
	41	Drowning
	39	Falls
	6	Medical X-rays
Drinking coffee	6	
Using oral contraceptives	5	
Drinking diet sodas	2	

effect. Certain conditions, such as alcoholism and schizophrenia, predispose people to isolation. Do unmarrieds become ill because they are isolated; or, are they isolated because they are ill? Most likely, it is not all one way or the other.

"Days Off Your Life" (table 1) does a good job of pointing out the relatively minor negative consequences of drinking coffee, using oral contraceptives, and consuming diet sodas. But table 1 does have its limitations. For example, the loss of 5 days of life expectancy from oral contraceptives is an average. For young, nonsmoking women the loss will be far less. (There is even some evidence that for this group of women, oral contraceptive use actually adds days to their lives by reducing the risk of ovarian and uterine cancer.) But for older women who are smokers, as we have seen, it's a different story. The days lost will be far more than 5.

A second approach to displaying health risks is "The Death Lottery" (table 2). It estimates how much of various activities are required to increase one's chances of dying, by one in a million, in any given year. Traveling 150 miles by car will do it. So will smoking 1.4 cigarettes, traveling 6 minutes in a canoe, living 2 months in an average stone or brick building, or eating 100 charcoal-broiled steaks, according to an article in *Technology Review* that analyzed daily risks.

An interesting perspective can be gained from going down the list and comparing different activities. One thing to note, however, is that some of these activities are associated with health problems other than those listed. Cigarette smoking, for example, is destructive to many systems in the body. In addition to cancer and heart disease, it significantly predisposes a person to emphysema and chronic bronchitis. Similarly, exposure to benzopyrene is not the only problem related to eating charcoal-broiled steaks; there are added risks from extra calories and concentrated fat intake. In these instances the risk is understated.

But overall, "The Death Lottery" provides a perspective that otherwise is difficult to grasp when we consider risk factors one at a time.

A third way of viewing health risks relates to the actual odds of adverse consequences. At a time when health hype insists on exaggerating our chances of catastrophe, "Risk Roulette" (table 3) puts the real numbers in front of us and provides a badly needed perspective.

Seeing these various odds for death laid out in descending order gives us a perspective that is difficult to capture any other way. So often we are faced with evaluating the seriousness of an isolated risk. When the numbers are seen in comparison to events and activities with which we are relatively familiar, the numbers take on new

Table 2. The Death Lottery

Activities Increasing Your Yearly Chances of Dying by One in a Million

Activities	Causes of Death
Smoking 1.4 cigarettes	Cancer, heart disease
Drinking 0.5 liter of wine	Liver cirrhosis
Eating 100 charcoal-broiled steaks	Cancer from benzopyrene
Eating 40 tablespoons of butter	Liver cancer (aflatoxin B)
Traveling 150 miles by automobile	Accident
Flying 1,000 miles by jet	Accident
Flying 6,000 miles by jet	Cancer from cosmic radiation
Traveling 10 miles by bicycle	Accident
Traveling 6 minutes by canoe	Accident
Living 2 months with a cigarette smoker	Cancer, heart disease
Living 2 months in average stone or brick building	Cancer from natural radioactivity
Living 2 months in Denver	Cancer from cosmic X-ray
Living 2 days in Boston or New York	Air pollution
Living 50 years within 5 miles of nuclear power plant	Cancer from accidental radiation release

meaning. It's instructive to compare the risk of merely being alive at various ages with other risks. Being age 35, for example, carries about the same risk as sport parachuting for a year. Notice that a year's worth of hang gliding—which I suspect many of us consider a dangerous sport—carries considerably less risk than undergoing elective hysterectomy. Hysterectomies are not innocuous procedures.

These various portrayals give some touchstones for roughly comparing health risks. They help clarify the big picture, and if we have the big picture in place, filling in the details becomes easier.

Table 3. Risk Roulette—Chances of Dying

Activity or Status	Chances of Dying
Age 65	1/39 per year
Motorcycling	1/50 per year
Aerial acrobatics (planes)	1/200 per year
Age 45	1/205 per year
Age 35	1/465 per year
Sport parachuting	1/500 per year
Elective hysterectomy	1/500 per event
Fire fighting	1/1,250 per year
Hang gliding	1/1,250 per year
Reyes Syndrome (among children with colds or flu, *treated with aspirin*)	1/2,264 per event
Age 10	1/3,832 per year
Hunting	1/33,333 per year
Pertussis immunization (permanent neurological damage)	1/330,000 per event
Polio immunization (Vaccine-polio from first oral dose)	1/520,000 per event
Commercial airplane trip	1/814,000 per trip
Lightning	1/2,000,000 per year
Automobile trip	1/4,000,000 per trip

Points to Remember

1. Accept the fact that there is some risk involved in everyday living.

2. Develop a tolerance for ambiguity. You'll need it. The facts are not all in.

3. Don't let health hype's love for the dramatic overly influence

you. It's the little things in life that kill us unexpectedly and early.

4. Watch out for the dread factor. Like the media, we overestimate the dangers of the unusual and the not-so-well understood.

5. When considering health facts, look for alternative ways of interpreting them. It helps in the understanding.

6. Don't automatically assume that modifying a risk factor will reduce the likelihood of a disease. Sometimes it does, sometimes it doesn't.

7. As much as possible, keep health risks in perspective. With headlines fighting you all the way, it's a tough job.

▶ ▶ ▶ ▶ ▶

I have never seen such an aggressive campaign as the "oat people" versus those of us who want a breakfast we can swallow.

They're everywhere. You can't turn on the television set without an oat disciple putting it to the guy who just wants to sit down and enjoy his sweet roll.

—Erma Bombeck,
    "Oat Bran Eaters Are Grim Reapers"
    August 20, 1989

▶ ▶ ▶ ▶ ▶ ▶ ▶ ▶

CHAPTER FOUR

Health News Tango

Decked out in its most scientific and up-to-date garb, health hype sweeps us off our feet by dancing around the facts, moving side to side, backward then forward, and jumping on the most profitable bandwagon. Never mind that its half-truths step on our toes; it is whispering sweet ambiguous nothings in our ears, and we don't want the dance to end for anything.

Health News Razzmatazz

Much of what is called "health" news is not news in the usual sense of the word. The problem in a nutshell is this: the American public wants to read, hear, and view more and more about health. When networks and newspapers survey their customers for what kind of information they want, health is consistently right at the top of the list. The media discovered some time ago, however, that what the public wants when it says "health information" is not the facts. We want lighter fare: health tips and speculations about the keys to beauty, fitness, and long life. So, the predictable has happened. Health news has mutated into a style-fashion-nutrition-food-fitness category with the accent on self-improvement. Health news has moved over to the entertainment section.

Once we understand this change, *why* certain items are chosen as "newsworthy," and how they are presented, becomes more understandable. No longer is the object to get the facts and present them objectively. That would be much too boring. The accent shifts to getting the item first and presenting it in its most dramatic, eye- or ear-catching form. Health news becomes health hype.

The media's fascination with health hype stems from the fact that it sells and sells and sells. The public wants it; the public gets it. It is a fortunate development for the media for this reason: with only a few notable exceptions, journalists and reporters are ill prepared to report health news in the traditional sense of news reporting. The image of a corps of specially trained health journalists and commentators out there critically poring over medical research reports to bring us the news is largely fiction. Most reporters assigned to health have little if any background in the health sciences or in research methodology. Typically, health-reporting assignments arise because nothing of greater interest is going on at the city desk or in the world of fashion, or whatever other area the reporter usually covers.

So the scene at most medical press conferences is predictable. Instead of assertive, well-prepared questioners skillfully working to get the facts and analyze them, more often than not reporters are passive and uncritically copying down what they are being told. Most of them are not technically knowledgeable enough to ask the right questions. Terminology itself is a major hurdle. It's difficult to ask illuminating questions if what you are hearing is in a foreign language. As for analyzing research design, forget it. For the most part, this goes unquestioned.

Imagine for a moment a White House press conference covered by sports reporters or journalists who generally write for the food and style sections of the newspaper. An equally inappropriate situation occurs daily with respect to the coverage of health news. Several years ago the American Council on Science and Health undertook a review of thirty periodicals that routinely carried articles on health. One out of three was found to be "inconsistent and unreliable." It reminds me of Mark Twain's comment: "Be careful about reading health books; you may die of a misprint." Fortunately, the errors in health reporting rarely lead to death; but, much of what is characterized as "health news" is misleading information.

Health News as Soap Opera

Television soap operas have developed a massive following extending even onto college campuses. (In fact, the popularity of the "soaps" has become such that a synopsis of the latest week's soap opera events has become essential reading among many fans.) There is now a "health news" equivalent to the soaps. Each week's episode is taken from one of the world's prestigious medical journals such as the *New England Journal of Medicine* and the *Journal of the*

American Medical Association. Many of the articles contained in these weekly publications are highly technical reports of medical research. While serving as important communications to other researchers and health-care professionals, they often report statistical findings that have no practical significance. These articles report research that, when further pursued, more often than not will lead down a blind alley. This is the way of science.

Until health hype discovered them, these technical research reports went largely unnoticed by the public. Now they have become part of a weekly ritual. The evening before official release, advance copies are made available to the media. The reports are hurriedly (and uncritically) translated into headlines for mass distribution the following day. This is how technical medical reports instantaneously become popular press items around the world.

Dr. Arnold Relman, editor of the *New England Journal of Medicine,* has criticized the media for the overcoverage of studies appearing in his own journal. "By and large, our content gets a lot of exposure—sometimes more than is warranted. Not in every issue, every week are there really newsworthy developments that merit a lot of attention. It's information that's of interest to the profession—not necessarily to the public," he told *Medical World News* (June 25, 1984).

There are two serious problems with the weekly "media watch" of medical research. One pertains to selection. Clearly, the selection criterion is entertainment value rather than scientific importance. This is why major advances are often overlooked and relatively insignificant findings are headlined. It's the topic that matters, not the design of the study, the strength of the finding, or its long-range importance. Given a choice between the study of a new weight-losing medication or the discovery of a new viral replication mechanism, "weight loss" will be the overwhelming choice most of the time. Why? Because it's something the consumer can relate to. It's much more sexy and salable. It won't matter that the reported weight loss is minimal and the side effects considerable. The relentless bias in favor of entertainment chitchat helps transform health news into fiction.

There's a second problem. Little attention is paid to context. Good newspapers and network news departments would never dream of reporting major breaking news without putting the unfolding events into context. Reporting medical research without reference to similar studies and without representing contrasting views is equally unacceptable. If the intention is to objectively report health news, current standards are woefully inadequate. (If entertainment is the goal, which it seems to be much of the time, the requirements are less exacting.)

The reading, listening, and viewing publics are titillated by reports from prestigious medical journals. So the media obliges. It glosses over the complicated and laborious nature of medical research. It downplays the fact that many of the results will turn out to be false starts and it readily fashions health suggestions from second-order statistical findings. Health news becomes "health tips"!

A case in point. In January 1988 the *Journal of the American Medical Association* carried a report on the medical treatment of "photo-aged" skin. A research team at the University of Michigan applied tretinoin cream (Retin-A) to the forearms and faces of thirty patients for sixteen weeks. They found twenty-nine of the thirty patients showed some reduction in "fine wrinkling" of the skin. The journal itself started the ball rolling with an editorial entitled, "At Last! A Medical Treatment for Skin Aging." The author maintained that after years when all the cosmetics industry had to sell was hope, now with the publication of the Michigan study, a "new age had dawned." That was enough for the media. They had their breakthrough health news story: old skin made young again.

In Los Angeles and Miami, drugstores sold out of Retin-A. "It's a bombshell," is the way one Miami pharmacist described the event. The *Los Angeles Times* (January 26, 1988) reported that even wholesalers ran out of stock. The manufacturer of Retin-A, Ortho Pharmaceutical Corporation, was forced to ration its supplies. It was all very good for business. The stock of Johnson & Johnson, the parent company, had run up six points as word spread of the impending medical journal report.

Retin-A is a prescription drug, but this appeared to present no real obstacle to patients anxious to make the wrinkles go away. Druggists commented on the willingness of doctors to sign prescriptions for an unapproved use of Retin-A. (In fact, the U.S. Food and Drug Administration had not even received an *application* for official clearance.)

Let's take a closer look at the basis for all the excitement: a single study of thirty patients for sixteen weeks. The result was limited to a reduction in fine wrinkles. Retin-A is an irritating substance. It causes skin inflammation and mild swelling in more than 90 percent of patients. (In fact, some dermatologists familiar with Retin-A have claimed that the disappearance of fine wrinkles is merely the result of swelling, which smoothes out the skin.) The study gives no information on how long the effect lasts. Will the medication have to be used for life? If so, will there be long-term adverse consequences? Even more basic, if the study is repeated will the same results be found?

The report on Retin-A for photo-aged skin was intriguing but very preliminary. The practical implications remain unclear—but not for the millions of Americans who (thanks to health hype) had been presented with a medical breakthrough via the media.

The popular audience for *real* health news is actually small. What the public wants is precisely what health hype so ably delivers, as it titillates, dazzles, and above all entertains. Clever wording is used to transform statistical findings into tantalizing health prescriptions. Researchers are described as having discovered factors that "may cause" heart disease or "are linked to" cancer or "may" play a role in preventing depression.

Researchers *Tie* Aluminum to Alzheimer's Disease

Sugar *May* Cause Heart Attacks

Aspirin *Connected* to Reyes Syndrome

Selenium *Might* Extend Life

Milk *May* Lower Risk of Cancer

High-Potassium Diet *Can* Combat Stroke

These cheat phrases allow headline writers to materialize health facts from statistical vapors.

Health Hype Horrors

Medical research taken out of context has led to far-reaching mistakes, as James Mills described in an article in the *Journal of the American Medical Association*. An earlier article in the same journal described a statistical association between the use of spermicidal agents around the time of conception and the subsequent development of congenital defects in the infant. The authors were careful to note: "The results should be considered tentative until confirmed by other data." Their note of caution was ignored. This "preliminary" report was picked up by the media and, eventually, by lawyers and treated as established fact.

Pregnant women who had used spermicidals around the time of conception became alarmed, and spermicide manufacturers were sued. To its credit, the *Journal of the American Medical Association* published a follow-up editorial reiterating the tentative nature of the findings. Following this a number of negative studies appeared in other journals, and the Food and Drug Administration determined through a series of hearings that the evidence was insufficient to even merit a warning label on spermicidals.

But the damage had been done. A major spermicide manufacturer lost a $4.7-million suit, and others face similar lawsuits. This is despite an official statement by the Food and Drug Administration that spermicides *do not* cause birth defects.

The "toxic shock scare" of 1980 represents another example of health fiction's capacity for irrevocable damage. Tremendous publicity was given to a serious condition of fever and shock (severe drop in blood pressure), mainly in younger women. Toxic Shock Syndrome (TSS), as the condition was to become popularly known, most often occurred in association with menstruation and the use of vaginal tampons. As is so often the case, uncovering the facts about this condition took a while. Each time a new piece of the puzzle was found, however, the popular press picked it up, and it became the whole story. At first tampons were the cause of this major killer. Period, case closed! This was the story in 1980, a year during which 4.4 billion tampons were sold in the United States but only 890 cases of TSS were reported with 42 deaths. (Even then, it should have been obvious that there was more to the story since the vast majority of women using tampons were not developing TSS.)

The story changed. The culprit was not *all* tampons, just those using a particular superabsorbent material. Protesting the weak evidence, Procter & Gamble wrote off $75 million for the 1982 recall of its Rely brand, and Playtex was slapped with a $11.2-million judgment involving a TSS death allegedly caused by a Playtex polyacrylate tampon. By 1985 all tampons made of polyacrylate (superabsorbent fiber) were withdrawn from the market. This was despite the fact that in 1984 (with tampon sales at $4.2 billion) the number of deaths from TSS had dropped to 4.

It is now clear that TSS is not caused by tampons per se. A far more likely candidate is infection by an endotoxin-producing strain of bacteria known as *Staphylococcus aureus.* Other toxins may be involved as well. TSS occurs in men and in nonmenstruating women. In fact one report found that this latter group has a death rate from TSS five times greater than do menstruating women. Roughly 6 percent of all adults harbor the bacterium capable of causing TSS. *Medical World News* reported in January 1987 that to the extent that the composition of tampons plays a role in TSS, according to the Center for Disease Control, it is probably a matter of overall absorbency rather than the particular kind of material used.

Despite the scare of 1980, TSS never came close to being a major killer, and the vilification of the manufacturers of superabsorbent tampons was premature and excessive. Health hype can do serious damage.

Health Reporter Blues

It would be unfair to ignore the small cadre of excellent medicine and science reporters. Year after year they skillfully pursue the reporting of health news as consummate professionals. But no matter how extensive a reporter's background and experience, assessing the validity and relative importance of developments in medicine and the health sciences is a tough assignment.

Despite its widespread popularity, health is not a favorite "hard news" item among news editors and producers. In a series of interviews with journalists, Dr. Jay Winsten, director of Harvard's Center for Health Communication, heard a recurrent theme about the fine line between exaggerated prose and copy that will never make it into print. One of the journalists commented: "We have to almost overstate, we have to come as close as we can within the boundaries of truth to a dramatic, compelling statement. A weak statement will go no place." Motivated by a driving ambition to make page one, these journalists clearly were familiar with being stuck between the rock and hard place of health reporting. It's a tricky business. When "strong" statements overshoot their mark, they become health fictions.

Peggy Eastman, a widely published health and science writer, described the problem to me. Reporters must *sell* editors on stories. If the editor doesn't bite, the story's dead. So the reporter constantly walks a tightrope between presenting the facts of the story and jazzing it up enough to convince the editor it will be a winner. Eastman has catalogued some of the responses she has received from editors about health stories in progress:

"Is this a cure for cancer or isn't it?"

"Cut all this stuff about beta-carotene. Make it simple: if people eat a lot of carrots, they won't get cancer."

"This story isn't exciting. Write something about the artificial heart."

There are plenty of editors and television and radio news directors who scoff at health stories carried in the *National Enquirer* while pushing for their own brand of health sensationalism.

Reverse Health Hype

Granted, the task of reporting AIDS has not been easy. It's a subject loaded with strong emotions, ugly politics, and lots of scientific unknowns. But there can be no doubt that AIDS is one of the most important health news stories of this century. While the press is adamant (as well it should be) about its first-amendment rights, with respect to AIDS, it didn't seem nearly as concerned about exercising them. Randy Shilts, in his outstanding book *And the Band Played On,* chronicles a strange, self-imposed silence on the part of the press during the first three years of the AIDS epidemic. Not once during that time did the annual Associated Press poll of editors and broadcasters turn up AIDS as one of the top-ten news stories. It finally made the list in 1985 after the death of Rock Hudson. Similarly, until the actor's death, no member of the White House press corps had asked (at least publicly) a single question about AIDS. By that time there had been twelve thousand reported cases of AIDS in the United States and six thousand deaths. AIDS stories in major print publications more than tripled in the first six months after Hudson's death. Why?

Undoubtedly, some of the reluctance to cover AIDS related to concern about "good taste." Many editors and producers who asked themselves, "Would our readers [or listeners or viewers] like to read this at the breakfast table?" answered, "No." They were afraid of squeamishness on the part of the consumer. When finally the subject of AIDS was broached, for some time the press relied upon a certain anesthetic language ("intimate body contact" and "exchange of bodily fluids"), even when these terms were clearly inadequate for the task at hand. Steve Findlay (now with *U.S. News & World Report*) related how initially in the reporting of AIDS for *USA Today*, he made readers guess what was going on rather than simply saying "anal intercourse."

With respect to AIDS, health hype operated in reverse, keeping the emerging tragedy out of our consciousness for as long as it could.

Medical Science Soft Shoe

Several years ago when I became interested in the subject of health fact vs. fiction, initially I assumed the latter was the exclusive product of the media. It was fashionable at the time (and still is) to blame the media for whatever was wrong. If you thought you weren't getting the facts, it was the journalists and commentators not doing their jobs. They whitewashed their stories or blew them all out of proportion. They were too naive or jaded, too simplistic or biased. It was all pretty convenient, the media was at fault.

It wasn't long, however, before I realized that this explanation for health fiction was not the whole story. The media had at least two other major partners.

If you ever bring up the subject with a group of reporters they immediately become defensive. They are quick to point out how medical researchers call press conferences at the drop of a hat to publicize self-serving, trivial findings. There is some truth in this.

Not too long ago, medical researchers seemed hesitant to get mixed up with the media. They were almost reluctant to publicize their work, for fear of being misquoted and having their results misinterpreted. After all, they said, their work could speak for itself when it appeared in professional journals. No more. Times have changed. Why? In one word: competition.

Media exposure can provide a winning edge in medical science.

Most medical researchers live or die through the research grant. It is their life blood, and in recent years it has become scarce. Less funds for more researchers have given impetus to the publicity-seeking researcher. Publicity has become a requirement, a fact of research life, actively encouraged by public relations offices in universities, hospitals, and medical technology corporations.

The press conference has become a widely used publicity tool. If researchers, especially those from prestigious institutions, call a press conference, the media is captive. Journalists and commentators cannot run the risk of being "scooped," so they show up. But they are at a distinct disadvantage since, as we have seen, seldom do they have the time, inclination, or background to prepare themselves. Instead, they rely on the researcher's appraisal of his or her own work. This is often the sole basis for identifying a "breakthrough" medical news story.

Here is an example of how the press conference can be commandeered and "used" by medical researchers. The March 8, 1985, issue of the *Journal of the American Medical Association* carried a report by Stanford researchers entitled, "Coffee Intake and Elevated Cholesterol and Apolipoprotein B Levels in Men." The journal article itself is cautiously presented. The authors studied seventy-seven middle-aged men and found a correlation between drinking two to three cups of coffee a day and a raised level of serum cholesterol as well as apolipoprotein B, a substance "thought to be more directly involved with atherosclerotic process than is the total amount of cholesterol in plasma." The authors carefully pointed out that other studies, some with much larger samples, contradicted their own, and that their study in no way established that coffee causes heart disease. This is what was said in the journal article. The press conference was another thing.

It was convened in a much more grandiose manner, as though a major medical discovery had been made. In doing so, the researchers were able to elicit far more attention for their modest results than was merited. The media responded with national exposure. *USA Today* carried the headline, "The Heart Risk for Coffee-drinking Men." Chalk up one more for the contribution of medical scientists to the art of health hoopla.

The press conference has become a way for researchers to make an "end run" around their own studies. This is how it is done: The results are written up strictly adhering to the constraints of research protocol. If the paper is accepted by a scientific journal, it appears in this cautiously worded form. But if the same researcher is in a press conference, the rules don't apply. What's said may depart dramatically from the results of the study itself. Microphones can be intimidating. They also can be intoxicating. They can seduce researchers into speaking far beyond what they legitimately can say.

Another case in point is far more serious. On October 29, 1985, three French scientists announced that cyclosporine, a drug currently used to prevent rejection of transplanted organs, would halt the growth of the AIDS virus. The basis for their announcement was *six* AIDS patients whom they had treated with cyclosporine and followed for *one week*. Never mind that cyclosporine, like the AIDS virus itself, *suppresses* the immune system and, at least theoretically, is a highly unlikely treatment. Never mind that no actual study was done; there was no control group, no protocols. Overlook the brief duration of the observation time and the fact that there were only six patients.

The media, much to the chagrin of other French researchers, carried the story around the world. Brief disclaimers, when they were included, were no match for large, eye-catching headlines. On October 30, 1985, the *Los Angeles Herald Examiner* put the story on page one—"The War on AIDS: French Announce Dramatic Treatment"—and followed it with a longer Associated Press story. On page fifteen, for the reader who stuck with the story, a few critical remarks from other scientists were woven into the story. Too little, too late.

More importantly, the subsequent real news story went unreported: how three French scientists, in a rush to make a medical coup, had prematurely announced a major breakthrough on the flimsiest of evidence. Within a matter of days, three of the six patients had died. More realistically, the story should have been headlined: "Three French Scientists Make Unsubstantiated Claim for AIDS Treatment."

Press conferences increasingly are being used by medical scientists to editorialize beyond their research findings. In this setting, there's a tendency to overstate results of narrowly defined research.

Personal opinions creep in. Hard evidence is displaced by educated guesses, which in turn become the basis for the next morning's "health news."

Riding Health All the Way to the Bank

Health fiction means profits. The marketplace is always on the lookout for another best-selling item. As the health benefits of various lifestyle changes are extolled, corporations and entrepreneurs wait and watch. Once it's clear a certain item has "legs" (is going to be around for awhile), store shelves quickly fill with the products alleged to bring us good health. The commercial world is the third major partner in the health news tango.

A look at today's advertising sections makes it abundantly clear that merchandisers believe health sells. So much so, it is difficult at times to distinguish between a promotional ad and a health message. The other day in the grocery store, I noticed that the Kellogg's All-Bran cereal box carried the salutation "To Your Health," with the imposing subtitle: "Preventative Health Tips from the National Cancer Institute."

The copy goes on to say: "Eat high fiber foods." Further down, the consumer is advised to write for the free "Cancer Prevention" booklet. At the bottom of the message/ad is a picture of Kellogg's All-Bran, labeled: MAXIMUM FIBER ALL-BRAN. That cereal box illustrates how commercial interests serve as a "flywheel" to perpetuate preliminary health findings regardless of whether or not they are confirmed.

The case for fiber in the prevention of cancer has been overblown. It is by no means established that if you start wolfing down large amounts of fiber (Kellogg's or any other brand), you can count on a lower risk of stomach or colon cancer, diabetes, gallstones, or irritable bowel syndrome. Furthermore, the adverse effects of ingesting lots of fiber have not been adequately portrayed. For many people loading up on bran quickly leads to distension, flatulence, and abdominal discomfort. Excess bran may also carry out of the body excessive amounts of essential nutrients. But these are the things you do not see, as everybody jumps on what a 1987 *Lancet* article called the "bran wagon."

When corporate America rushes in, it's like etching the message in granite. The fiber story (encouraged by the finest advertising corporate millions can buy) will be around for a long time, even if contradictory evidence should turn up. Market share does not come easily, and it's not going to be relinquished just because of a few new facts.

Consider another example of commercial health hype, designed to sell a product known as "Vittel, a California naturally sparkling mineral water." A full-page ad in the *Pacific Southwest Airline Magazine* is captioned with the provocative question: CAN A WATER ACTUALLY INCREASE YOUR STAMINA?"

Then comes the zinger: "MAGNESIUM IS THE STAMINA MINERAL."

And if you don't question that line, the rest seems logical:

Poor diet, stress and exercise all deplete magnesium. And if you're going to burn it, you've got to return it.

INTRODUCING VITTEL.

Of course proclaiming magnesium as the "stamina mineral" is purely a leap of faith, as are the assumptions that most of us eat so poorly, are stressed so severely, or exercise so vigorously that we "burn up" all our body's magnesium. But, all in all, a clever promotion, illustrating health's marvelous marketing possibilities.

For another example we can turn to a recent advertisement for Tylenol. This effort takes "the most trusted name in pain relief" and tries to make it the most trusted name in stress reduction. Quite a leap!

I do not have to tell you how overworked the concept of stress has become in the 1980s. As Public Health Enemy Number One, stress has spawned relaxation clinics, books, and seminars as well as a host of self-help aids. So the makers of Tylenol understandably have decided to get a piece of the stress-reduction business, a new and lucrative market.

The full-page ad is captioned at the top:

STRESS

AND HOW TO LIVE WITH IT

The ad first provides a brief overview of stress. Some stress is good, but if you get too much it becomes distress. If so, what can you do about it? You can listen to music, take a walk, or just talk to someone.

So far, so good. But you're probably wondering how the ad gets around to the idea of taking Tylenol. The answer is, circuitously. It points out that if you have too much stress you may get stomach disturbances or a *headache*, in which case you might consider aspirin, but that might not be such a good idea because aspirin—even buffered aspirin—might further upset your stomach. Then with a great light touch, the ad drives home its message: "You may feel that, as life becomes more stressful, it is better to stay away from aspirin altogether. For this reason, you might choose an acetaminophen product like Tylenol."

Don't think for a second that the makers of Tylenol have a corner on the stress-reduction market. The March 1986 issue of *Consumer Reports* carried an article entitled "The Vitamin Pushers." In a section called "Hype about Stress," the writers review vitamin preparations sold as protection against stress. Sears's Puritan's Pride Stress Formula is promoted on the basis that "active lives subject us to considerable stress. . . . All these types of stress increase your body's needs for vitamins." I. Magnin department stores recommend Clientele Stress Control Nutrients if "you find yourself drained from everyday events." A major wholesaler of vitamin ingredients, Hoffmann-LaRoche, advertises that "if you drink, smoke, diet or happen to be sick, you may be robbing your body of vitamins." Ayerst Laboratories gets right to the point by declaring that "just being alive is stressful" and recommends Beminal Stress Plus.

Vitamins, and mineral supplements as well, are marvelously flexible products. With a little imagination, you can promote them for just about anything. And that is exactly what has happened. Every once in a while, however, the claims are so outrageous that a regulatory agency gets involved.

In October 1987, Great Earth International, a nationwide chain of food-supplement stores based in southern California, was forced by the Federal Trade Commission to sign a consent decree to stop advertising "TriAmino Plus P.M." The company had promoted this product as an overnight weight-loss remedy. "Lose while you snooze" was the advertising pitch. Good-bye diet books! Great Earth International claimed that TriAmino Plus P.M. stimulated the production of growth hormone, which, in turn, burned up fat. Fascinating idea, but false.

Under the decree the company agreed to refrain from making

specific claims about its product. Several months later, a manager of one of the Great Earth stores reported that sales were still strong for TriAmino Plus P.M. He attributed this to the advertising of similar products by other companies and to health magazine articles.

For every commercial interest that gets its hands slapped, hundreds go undisciplined. The health craze has been a tremendous boon for many commercial interests, responsible and unresponsible alike. And what could be better, the hucksters reason, than making a buck off of what makes people "healthier."

Money Talks

Cigarettes are a serious health hazard, we all know. They are also one of the most heavily advertised products in America. These two facts create a serious conflict for various publications that provide health coverage. The revenues from cigarette advertising are a sizable part of their income. If their coverage includes the negative consequences of smoking, cigarette manufacturers will not be pleased. Likely they will take their advertising dollars elsewhere. What is the answer? For many magazines it has been to take the money and "overlook" the health consequences of smoking.

One investigator, after examining coverage devoted to cigarettes and cancer over a seven-year period in the 1970s, concluded that "advertising revenue can indeed silence the editors of American magazines." He had been unable to find a single article clearly describing the negative health consequences of cigarette smoking.

A few American magazines have resolved this dilemma by refusing to accept any cigarette advertising. (This has been true of *Reader's Digest, Good Housekeeping*, the *New Yorker*, and the *Washington Monthly*.) Most magazines, however, have not taken this course, and it shows in the paucity of their comments.

In his 1984 book *The Smoke Ring*, Peter Taylor refers to a 1982 survey conducted by the American Council on Science and Health. *Ms.* magazine, while receiving $500,000 in cigarette advertising money (15 percent of its total revenue) ran *no* articles on the health hazards of smoking. This was a particularly striking omission given the magazine's extensive coverage of health matters. Cigarette smoking is responsible for 300,000 to 400,000 deaths a year, which is many times the number of deaths caused by all the illegal drugs combined. *Ms.* portrays the dangers of street drugs but doesn't run a single article on cigarettes, which have singlehandedly drawn lung cancer alongside breast cancer in a race to become the leading killer of women. Oversight? No way.

Other magazines showing a similar pattern included *Redbook, Mademoiselle, Parade,* and *Time.*

Remember, health fiction works both ways: it can exaggerate or it can underplay. The result is the same: a serious distortion of facts.

Points to Remember

1. Health news is more like entertainment than like regular news.

2. If you think there is a large corps of well-trained health reporters, you are wrong. (My apologies to the notable few who are excellent.)

3. Mark Twain's comment still holds: "Be careful about reading health books; you may die of a misprint."

4. The *Journal of the American Medical Association* and the *New England Journal of Medicine* are outstanding medical journals. That does not mean that everything that appears in them is newsworthy.

5. Watch out for cheat phrases: "Soup *May* Cause Purple Hair," "Thinking *Linked* to Aging," or "Sex *Tied* to Cancer."

6. Remember one editor's words to his reporter: "Is this a cure for cancer or isn't it?" There is a lot of ambiguity in health matters, but you won't hear much about it. Gray is not a popular journalistic color.

7. Health fiction works both ways: It exaggerates and it underplays, depending on where the money is.

8. There are no guarantees at press conferences called to announce "medical breakthroughs." Trivia turns up there about as often as important findings do.

9. Some of the best health hype is in advertising.

10. You can get *too much* bran!

▸ ▸ ▸ ▸ ▸

By now it [the public] suspects that what is banned today is likely to be administered in all the best clinics tomorrow. It has learned to invert the findings where necessary, to discount the permanence of any of them, to make the unwholesome, illogical best of whatever it is told. Nixon is back. Everything is back. Twinkies will be back. They will be telling us to put more salt on them.

—Meg Greenfield, *Newsweek, June 25, 1984*

CHAPTER FIVE

▸ ▸ ▸ ▸ ▸ ▸ ▸ ▸

Fickle Medicine

Doctors are not always right. They're only human, and, as such, are bound to make mistakes. But more important, they make black and white decisions from medicine's very gray palette, practicing medicine based on existing knowledge that is not always correct or complete. They really have no choice. Whether they have—or think they have—all the answers or not, the patients will keep coming in. It's a sad fact that many of today's recommended treatments and procedures will be discovered to be ineffective or even harmful tomorrow. Medicine is fickle.

Sleight-of-Hand Medicine

Not too many years ago women were told to have Pap smears annually. Then experts got together and decided this was unnecessary. The reasoning was that cervical cancer (the condition the Pap smear detects) progresses slowly. Even if it goes undetected for a few years, there's no real harm; it will still be curable. So the Pap smear recommendation was changed. The new guideline was more lenient: after two normal Pap smears, a woman could go for three years before being screened again. Her risk would be no greater. A few years passed, and experts (perhaps the same ones) met again. Things had changed. Cases of cervical cancer seemed to show more rapid progression. The cause was unclear. Some felt it was due to an increased spread of the infectious agents involved in sexually transmitted diseases. Perhaps these were playing a part in the accelerated development of cervical cancer. Regardless, the experts agreed: the present guideline was not adequate. It was not enough to have a Pap smear once every three years. The annual Pap smear was back in vogue.

Medical truth vacillates. Now you see it, now you don't. Consider, for example, the annual physical examination, characterized for years as essential to good health. Beginning in the early 1900s, physicians persuaded industrialists that having their employees show up for yearly examinations would keep down the number of sick days and even improve job performance. The annual health checkup was a must, particularly the doctor's physical examination.

When put to the test, however, the annual physical examination comes up short. People who have regular checkups do no better than those who do not. Neither their health status nor their life expectancy is improved. Perhaps one of the reasons is the lack of sensitivity of the physical examination. Overall, it is a fairly crude screening method, often unable to detect early disease. Today, routine physical examinations are out of vogue.

Ulcer Theories Come and Go

Just a few years ago the facts about peptic ulcers were pretty cut-and-dried. First of all, persons with this condition had definite psychological problems. They could not stand up to tough situations. They were overly susceptible to stress and, just beneath the surface, were dependent personalities. They were worriers, they had worried themselves into an ulcer.

After being told the psychological origins of their ulcers, patients were given a litany of things to do to relieve their symptoms. As they undertook a total psychological overhaul, they were also supposed to avoid all spicy foods. Chili, curry, salsa, and hot mustards were taboo. Bland food was the order of the day. The idea was that spicy foods somehow added to the corrosive effects of stomach acid.

And there was more. The food had to be taken in frequent feedings. The ulcer patient could no longer join up with the rest of the population for three meals a day. Instead, every two to three hours he or she was to eat a small serving. This was supposed to decrease the secretion of stomach acid. The most highly recommended food for these small feedings was milk, because it neutralized the acid—at least that was the theory.

There were other definite no-no's. No alcohol or caffeine. The person might as well have been drinking acid itself. When an ulcer patient failed to improve, it was thought that he was undisciplined. Clearly, he was not adhering to his anti-ulcer diet.

Just a few years later, most of this gospel about ulcer treatment has now been discredited. People who develop ulcers are believed to be genetically predisposed: they are *born* with a physiologic susceptibility. There is no "ulcer personality"; and, as for the role of stress, high-stress workers are no more likely to develop peptic ulcers than are laid-back workers. The anti-ulcer diet was a medical myth. People on bland diets do not heal ulcers faster than those who eat regular or even spicy foods. And frequent feedings not only do not reduce the amount of stomach acid, they actually increase it! Furthermore, although milk sometimes relieves peptic ulcer pain, it turns out to be a potent stimulus of gastric acid, while wine, beer, and caffeine do not cause a lot more acid secretion than other things we regularly eat.

If you look closely, these erroneous ulcer treatments were all "reasonable" ideas, but they were sold and accepted as proven methods before being put to the test. Having now been critically examined, they are falling by the wayside and being recognized for what they are: medicine's own brand of health fiction.

Schizophrenigenic Families

For another example of fickle medicine, we can turn to psychiatry.

Schizophrenia is a tragic disease. In this country it affects roughly one out of every hundred persons. Contrary to popular belief, it is *not* a disorder of multiple personalities. Typically, it appears in late adolescence or early adulthood. Often the person begins to have hallucinations (hearing or seeing things that are not present and expressing bizarre thoughts). The person may sense he or she is the target of a sordid plot or is being subjected to strange influences over his or her mind. In between these psychotic episodes, the "schizophrenic" lives as a loner, having great difficulty relating to other people. He or she may laugh or cry at the wrong time and generally cannot socialize comfortably.

In the 1960s, the idea was advanced that schizophrenia was caused by disturbed family communications. The theory held that the "victim," caught in a web of contradictory communications, eventually went mad. For evidence the proponents of this theory pointed to the chaotic relationships often characterizing these families. The possibility that the reverse might be true—that schizophrenia might cause family disturbances rather than being caused by them—was overlooked in the selling of the "schizophrenigenic family." Consequently, for almost two decades, parents of schizophrenic children, at the same time they were confronted with their child's tragic condition, were blamed for causing it.

As E. Fuller Torrey describes in his book *Surviving Schizophrenia*, the condition is now thought to be a brain disease. It is not caused by parents who talk "crazy" to their children, a belief for which there never was really any substantial evidence. Nor is schizophrenia cured by getting families to talk differently. What is clear is that the guilt suffered by these parents was a painful and undeserved cost of psychiatric health fiction.

From time to time, conclusions based on unproven medical hunches prove devastating. Not only is the treatment ineffective, it is injurious in its own right. In *Matters of Life and Death: Risks vs. Benefits of Medical Care*, Stanford's Dr. Eugene Robin called these medically induced injuries "iatroepidemics."

Iatroepidemics occur when a reasonable treatment idea is accepted prematurely as medical fact. In the absence of scientific studies, it is successfully pitched to the medical profession and widely accepted. Once accepted, the false treatment becomes an entrenched medical myth. Eventually, usually only after an overwhelming amount of contradictory evidence accumulates, the prevailing practice is dethroned. The mistake is acknowledged and a new approach taken, but too late to benefit the victims who have gone before.

Radical Mastectomy

From the early 1900s until the 1970s, the surgical procedure known as radical mastectomy was *the* recommended treatment for cancer of the breast. In this operation, the breast is removed along with much of the surrounding soft tissue, including muscles of the chest. It is disfiguring, to say the least.

Radical mastectomy was introduced by a well-meaning surgeon who felt that it made good sense. He assumed that breast cancer always spread to the surrounding area; therefore, the more tissue removed, the greater the chances of survival. At that time (1907), not much was known about cancer other than that it was a killer. There were no proven alternative treatments. Radical mastectomy became the definitive treatment, largely based on one man's hunch. It was adopted without ever being compared to less radical surgery.

It was not until the 1950s that this mutilating operation was seriously questioned. By that time huge numbers of women had undergone this surgery, having been told that without it, they had virtually no chance of surviving their breast cancer. Faced with a choice between disfigurement and death, most women underwent the operation.

In 1955 another surgeon reported a small clinical trial in which he compared radical mastectomy to a procedure in which he removed only the cancer itself (lumpectomy) and followed this up with radiation therapy. The second group, far less disfigured, had fared as well as the first. Not unexpectedly, given the long reign of radical mastectomy, this alternative treatment was not accepted initially. Only after another twenty-five years and the accumulation of substantial comparative evaluation evidence, particularly from Europe, did lumpectomy and radiation become medically respectable and widely recommended for treatment of *localized breast cancer*.

As is so often the case in the aftermath of iatroepidemics, controversy lingers. Dr. Robin points out that some experts, mainly surgeons, claim that after fifteen or twenty years women treated with radical mastectomies show slightly higher survival rates than those receiving lumpectomies and radiation. He also makes this observation: "It is more or less a general rule of iatroepidemics that the specialist whose practice is being challenged—the one whose 'ox is gored'—leads the defense of the old practice."

In October of 1987 then First Lady Nancy Reagan was diagnosed as having breast cancer. She was confronted with the same decision thousands of women face each year. Should she have a mastectomy or should she opt for lumpectomy and radiation? She did not take long to decide. After conferring with her physicians, she chose a mastectomy. From the information made available, it appeared that she qualified equally as well for the other option. Having been detected early, her breast cancer was extremely small, well within the limits for lumpectomy combined with radiation. Still, Mrs. Reagan chose mastectomy.

We probably will never know how she arrived at her decision (and it really is no one else's business). But I cannot help wondering if it doesn't reflect the continuing difficulty in accepting the alternative approach. Put yourself in the place of the physicians advising Mrs. Reagan. They knew the decision would be publicized across the world almost instantaneously. They must have felt tremendous pressure to recommend the "tried and true." There was substantial evidence that a nonmastectomy would produce an equally advantageous outcome, but it was a "newer" treatment—not a conservative choice and not the one to recommend with all the world watching.

Regardless, the First Lady's choice probably set back considerably the acceptance of lumpectomy and radiation as the treatment for localized, early breast cancer.

Iatroepidemics in Progress

One of the more traumatic moments from my own childhood relates to having my tonsils removed. As I recall it now, I was kept in the dark about what was in store. I knew it had something to do with the sore throat I had been having. That was about it. In the hospital clinic, I was taken into a room and asked to lie down on an examining table. The doctor came in, and after a few pleasantries and reassurances that what was about to happen wouldn't hurt, everything went dark. Later, I was told this was the point at which a cloth soaked in an anesthetic was placed over my face. As I lay screaming, the doctor called to me to yell louder so they could hear me. (Apparently, so I would breathe in the anesthetic.) I obliged him, screaming at the top of my lungs. The next thing I remember was waking up with a very sore throat and an upset stomach. My tonsils had been removed.

For decades tonsillectomy was performed routinely on millions of children. Evidence now shows, at least in most cases, that this operation is unnecessary and may well be detrimental, since tonsils contribute to the body's defense against infections. And like any surgical procedure, tonsillectomy carries a degree of risk. There are complications, and in about one in fifteen thousand tonsillectomies, a child dies.

Tonsillectomy continues to be the single most common surgery performed on children. In the United States, some 400,000 tonsillectomies are done each year. In light of the evidence, why is this surgical procedure not on the decline? Simple. Because it is lucrative, and it is an established practice. (Once enshrined in medical officialdom, such practices have terrific staying power, especially when they favorably affect the practitioner's pocketbook.) But unless

Table 4. Medical/Procedures Review (Rand Corporation Study, 1987)

	Inappropriate	Equivocal	Total Questionable
Coronary arteriography	17.4%	8.5%	25.9%
Carotid endarterectomy	32.4%	32.3%	64.7%
Upper gastrointestinal tract endoscopy	17.2%	10.8%	28.0%

a child suffers from recurrent attacks of tonsillitis that fail to respond to antibiotics, tonsillectomy should be considered suspect.

Tonsillectomy is not the only procedure being overdone. In November 1987 a five-year study by the Rand Corporation was reported in the *Los Angeles Times* that claimed that thousands of medical/surgical procedures were being performed unnecessarily in this country each year. Using a panel of experts, the study reviewed three million patient records involving 819 physicians and 227 different hospitals. It focused on three specific procedures. The first was the surgical removal of blockages in the major arteries to the brain known as "carotid endarterectomy." The second was "coronary arteriography," a procedure that requires the introduction of a catheter into the heart for the purpose of injecting dye that can be visualized by X-ray. And the third was "upper gastrointestinal tract endoscopy," a diagnostic examination performed by passing a flexible, fiber-optic lighted tube into the gastrointestinal tract.

A rating system was devised to evaluate the procedures: If the potential benefits outweighed the possible dangers by a "sufficient degree," they were judged "appropriate"; if not, they were "inappropriate"; or in instances that were unclear, they were "equivocal" (see table 4).

Each of the procedures was rated as inappropriate or questionable in a sizable number of cases (no less than 25 percent). Carotid endarterectomy—a procedure with serious potential adverse consequences—showed the poorest rating. Almost a third were considered inappropriate and a similar number questionable.

The Rand study serves to remind us that there are fads in medicine and surgery. Once a procedure becomes established, it will likely be overused. You want to make certain you are not the person on whom it's being overused. If a medical/surgical procedure is recommended, you should never fail to ask this basic question: What do I have to gain and what do I have to lose? When you find out, make up your own mind.

Cesarean section is another overused surgery. At 24 percent of all deliveries, the cesarean rate in the United States is the world's highest. There has been a meteoric rise since 1970 when the rate was only 5.5 percent. The Public Citizen Health Research Group has estimated that fully half of the 906,000 cesareans performed in 1986 were unnecessary, according to a December 1987 report in *Medical World News.*

Even many obstetricians agree that the number of cesareans is excessive, although they often balk at the idea that the problem arises mainly because of the financial incentives involved. Income may well be one of the factors, but it is not the only one. Cesareans sometimes are done out of concern over being sued for malpractice. Another factor is the feelings of the patients themselves. Cesarean sections are preferred by some women, apparently even when there is no specific medical indication.

There are definite indications for a cesarean section. Used appropriately it is a valuable procedure, often benefiting both mother and infant. Major surgery of any kind, however, is not to be taken lightly. It carries its own set of risks.

Seeing without Glasses

Radial keratotomy was first developed in the Soviet Union in 1974, and five years later it was introduced in this country. Since then more than 175,000 have been performed. It's a simple eye surgery procedure for correcting nearsightedness (myopia). Using local anesthetic, an operating microscope, and a high-precision diamond knife, the ophthalmologist makes a dozen or so tiny incisions in the cornea, causing it to flatten. This shifts the focus of the visual image back onto the retina, allegedly restoring visual acuity to normal. The procedure takes five to ten minutes to complete. The eye is then patched for twenty-four hours and pain medication is prescribed for a few days. On the average, the cost runs about $1,500 but price wars seem to be common, with bargain rates appearing.

Radial keratotomy has been highly publicized as a problem-free alternative to glasses or contact lenses. Now that there has been time to evaluate it, the emerging story is not quite so rosy, according to a report in *Ophthalmology*.

Studies have raised serious questions about the consistency of results from this operation. There seems to be no guarantee that the two eyes will turn out to have the same visual acuity. Furthermore, the effectiveness of the operation is often less than that which is publicized. About four out of five people achieve only partial correction to 20/40. And in those cases where 20/20 is achieved, it often changes over time, eventually requiring the person to resort to lenses once again—sometimes as a result of having become farsighted! Other complications have surfaced, including long delays—up to four years—in healing. More rarely, persons have suffered serious eye infections, cataracts, retinal detachment, and even blindness.

Certainly, the final word is not in on radial keratotomy. But for the moment, caution is indicated. As is so often the case, this "breakthrough" has not lived up to its initial promises.

The Drug Epidemic

When people talk about the "drug problem," they usually mean illicit street drugs such as heroin, PCP, and "crack." Often overlooked is the modern epidemic of *prescribed drugs*. If I had to pick one current medical practice that most likely will be labeled an iatroepidemic in years to come, it would be the over-prescribing of medications.

There are two reasons. First, the number of persons receiving medications has become staggering. More and more of us take medication, and as we age we increasingly take more than our share. People over the age of sixty-five on the average consume twice as many medications as younger persons. Second, the medications themselves have become more potent. While that is good in some ways, it is bad in others: namely, their adverse side effects. Unfortunately, the scorekeeping for these negative drug reactions is extremely spotty, so the full damage of the prescription drug epidemic goes understated.

Every medication has a cost/benefit profile. All medications carry a degree of risk, albeit some considerably more than others. Unless there is a likely prospect of benefit, medications can be losing propositions.

Antibiotics are a good example. By this time you would think everyone would know that antibiotics do not work against the common cold or against most other viral infections for that matter. Right? Wrong! Antibiotics are one of the most misused drugs we have. When taken indiscriminately they endanger a person by wiping out normal bacteria and leaving the field vulnerable to attack by fungi and other opportunistic organisms. Several years ago a study showed that 40 percent of patients in the Johns Hopkins Hospital received at least one antibiotic that was not indicated. This is a particularly risky practice since the unwarranted use of antibiotics has a way of breeding "super bugs." These mean-spirited bacteria aggressively infect and are the devil to get rid of.

Medications can also have adverse consequences of their own. In fact, these consequences cause about one out of every ten hospital admissions. Additionally, once in the hospital, roughly one out of three patients becomes sick on medications they receive, according to a 1970 study in the *Journal of the American Medical Association*, entitled "Comprehensive Drug Surveillance."

Medications are problematic also in the deleterious effect they can have on one another. While computers may be able to keep up with the myriad of drug-drug combinations, mortal physicians are not equal to the task. The book *Pills, Profits and Politics,* by Milton Silverman and Philip Lee, describes a research investigation on prescriptions given out over twelve months to forty-two thousand patients that revealed that close to one out of ten had received potentially incompatible medications. The medications had either canceled each other out or, worse still, interacted to create a toxic effect. If you add the various over-the-counter drugs that people take on their own to the medications they receive from their doctors, the potential for "bad" combinations is considerable. It is estimated that roughly 5 percent of all hospital admissions in this country result from adverse drug reactions. Drugs—the legitimate kind—definitely can be hazardous to your health.

How High Is High?

One of the most effective health education campaigns in years has convinced us of the dangers of hypertension. Some sixty million

Americans are thought to harbor this "silent killer." Few of us have not heard or read about the importance of getting treatment to avoid premature strokes and heart attacks.

In the early 1980s the assistant secretary for health, Edward N. Brandt, Jr., reported to Congress that the evidence was clear: any degree of high blood pressure was bad and should be treated in order to prolong life. The stage was set.

A potential market of this magnitude quickly attracts attention. High blood pressure screening centers are everywhere, in supermarkets and drugstores. Electronic firms have created home-care kits to more easily alert consumers to this "silent killer." Physicians are poised with an impressive armamentarium of drugs obligingly served up by the pharmaceutical industry to combat even the slightest sign of high blood pressure.

But in the past few years, evaluation studies have turned up some troubling results, and experts now seriously question the wisdom of treating the mildest cases of hypertension. There is general agreement that drug treatment should be undertaken for individuals with diastolic blood pressures (the lower number) above 100. Additionally, if a person has several other risk factors for heart disease, such as smoking and high blood cholesterol, treatment is recommended for diastolic blood pressure above 90. Drug treatment is *not* indicated for diastolic pressures below 90. Beyond this, consensus falls apart. For the millions who do not have other heart risk factors and whose diastolic blood pressure is below 100 but above 90, they are on their own. This is the gray zone; the limbo area. But keep in mind the forces of the marketplace. They keep the drums beating for treating even the slightest touch of hypertension.

A person with mild hypertension trying to decide about treatment should keep a few facts in mind. First, the benefits. Dr. Edward Freis of the Veterans Administration Medical Center in Washington, D.C., provided the following analysis in the *New England Journal of Medicine*. A forty-five-year-old man with a diastolic pressure of 95 and no other risk factors who receives treatment that reduces his diastolic pressure to below 90 over a six-year period will lessen his chances of heart attack by one percent. A benefit, yes, but a modest one.

Now for the negatives. Going on medication for the rest of your life should not be taken lightly. Doctors' fees, medication costs, and the expense of laboratory tests over the years add up, not to mention the inconvenience of being a "chronic patient." In addition, hypertension medication (depending on which kind you take) has its share of untoward side effects. Fatigue, dizziness, sexual dysfunction—particularly impotence in men—and depression are common problems. A group of drugs known as "beta blockers" have become widely prescribed antihypertensive agents. A 1986 report in the *Journal of the American Medical Association* of a two-year study found that 20 percent of patients on beta blockers ended up depressed, women four times as often as men.

If you are one of those persons who has a "touch" of hypertension, you should not feel you are risking your life by not taking medication. But I warn you, those "silent killer" posters may give you trouble from time to time. Health hype can keep you awake at night. You just have to learn how to brush it off when its headlines do not apply to you. Keep in mind that people with mild hypertension often find that dietary changes and exercise bring down their blood pressure. These would seem prudent approaches to take before embarking on a treatment whose adverse side effects may outweigh its benefits.

Most important, do not accept a single blood pressure reading as unequivocal evidence of high blood pressure. Some people react stressfully to the very act of having their blood pressure taken. For these individuals, a mild elevation in their blood pressure reflects the stress of being in the presence of a doctor or nurse.

Researchers have coined the term "white-coat hypertension" to refer to a situation in which a person's blood pressure jumps up in the presence of a doctor. One recent study found that out of 292 patients thought to have borderline high blood pressure, 21 percent had "white-coat hypertension." Their blood pressure would rise in the doctor's office, but all through the rest of the day (as measured by a special twenty-four-hour blood pressure recorder worn on their arms) they had normal blood pressure. In this study most of the physicians taking blood pressures were men and most of the patients were women. The researchers feel that women may be more susceptible to this condition than men.

Given the recent emphasis on blood pressure monitoring, "high blood pressure" has become one of those diagnoses that has a way of getting attached to people whose conditions really don't warrant it. Make sure it doesn't happen to you. If you are truly hypertensive, your blood pressure will be significantly elevated on a number of occasions and in more than one setting.

Type A Behavior: Good or Bad

In the 1950s two doctors described a new way of categorizing people: Type A or Type B. If you were Type B, you were in luck. You were easygoing, relaxed, able to take things in stride, and (most important) unlikely to become a victim of heart disease. This was in contrast to Type A's. If you were one of these, you were a hard-driving workaholic, competitive, overly aggressive, and always racing against the clock. You were a walking heart attack waiting to happen. Independent of other risk factors, Type A's were twice as likely to get heart disease, so it was said.

Training programs were offered to remake Type A's into Type B's by getting these people off the race track; to have them mellow out and take things easier. For many Type A's it took a heart attack to drive the point home. The training programs were particularly popular with post–heart attack victims. They were conditioned to accept the folly of their ways as Type A's.

In the 1980s, however, the tide began to turn. Studies appeared that failed to confirm the increased risk for Type A's. These findings were fiercely rebutted by firm believers of Type A–Type B. But the contradictory evidence kept coming. Finally, in January 1988 a lead article appeared in the *New England Journal of Medicine* reporting what would have been unspeakable a few years earlier. The researchers studied 257 men from the original investigation that had given birth to the whole idea of Type A–Type B, comparing the rates of survival of the two types after they had had heart attacks. They discovered that Type A men had survived heart attacks better than Type B's.

The researchers conjectured that Type A men might cope better with the event of a heart attack. Perhaps they are more determined in sticking to medical treatment and changing their life-style. Whatever the reason, the fact that for Type A's the risk of dying after a heart attack was only 60 percent that of Type B's reminds us again of the fickle nature of medical truth. What's said today may not be ascribed to tomorrow. Count on it.

Cholesterol: A New Wrinkle

The same people who brought us the "definitive" cholesterol study (one of our chapter 2 nominees to the Health Hype Hall of Fame) have recently had to confront a troublesome finding.

For several years the cholesterol saga has been unfolding as a good-guy/bad-guy story. As the story goes, not all cholesterol is bad for us. Only the kind known as LDL. The other cholesterol, HDL, actually plays a protective role. The more the better. Some researchers were even beginning to suggest that measuring a person's cholesterol level was not good enough. What was really needed was to measure the ratio between the good and bad cholesterols. The higher the ratio (more HDL to LDL) the better. An intensive search had already begun to discover ways of selectively raising HDL levels. Exercise was being pushed. Ditto moderate alcohol consumption. Then the Russians messed things up.

A fifteen-year collaborative study between the United States and the Soviet Union produced results that did not fit the good-cholesterol / bad-cholesterol study line. "In a major challenge to the widely held belief that a 'bad' form of cholesterol contributes to heart disease while another form helps prevent it, U.S. and Soviet researchers have found that high levels of the supposedly 'good' cholesterol offer no such protection to middle-aged Soviet men and are associated with an increase in the overall death rate," the *Los Angeles Times* reported November 18, 1987. And there was more. Soviet men with extremely low cholesterol levels had a *higher* incidence of heart disease!

The same researchers who had aggressively pushed low-cholesterol diets for all Americans were left scratching their heads, reluctant to accept their new findings but having little alternative. Back to the drawing boards.

Despite its considerable triumphs, modern medicine does not have all the answers. What it firmly believes and confidently practices today may be destined for tomorrow's scrap heap. Looking back, the mistakes made in patient care are written off as the cost of medical progress; and while this may be the truth, it is not a very consoling explanation for the patients who have suffered.

The message should be clear: if you want to avoid becoming a research-and-development casualty, evaluate medical claims carefully.

Points to Remember

1. Medical truth is tentative, but seldom will you find it billed as such.

2. Medical truths that have become myths:
   Ulcer diets work.
   Mastectomy is the only treatment for breast cancer.
   Families cause schizophrenia.
   Tonsils are bad.

3. There is too much surgery in this country. If you are considering having it, make certain you stand to gain more than you lose. That is not always the case.

4. There are too many medications. Have a good reason for taking one.

5. The diagnosis of high blood pressure is in vogue. Before you accept that you've got it, have your blood pressure taken several times, preferably in different settings.

6. If you have suffered disparaging remarks about your Type A behavior, take heart—you may have the last laugh.

7. Believe what you want to about cholesterol. There is plenty of evidence for it!

▸ ▸ ▸ ▸ ▸

You may not find out anything about the case. Then say that he has an obstruction of the liver, and particularly use the word "obstruction," because they do not understand what it means, and it helps greatly that a term is not understood by the people.

—Arnold of Villanova,
thirteenth-century
surgeon

CHAPTER SIX

▸ ▸ ▸ ▸ ▸ ▸ ▸

When More Is Less—
The Pitfalls of Medical Testing

Granted, it seems perfectly logical to have a doctor give you the once-over, just to be on the safe side. After all, if there are any diseases or mean-tempered bacteria lurking about in your body, the medical tests will find them, and then you and your doctor can work on eradicating them.

But what if these medical tests are not accurate? Or are out-and-out false? Believe it or not, some medical tests cause more harm than good. In his book *Matters of Life and Death: Risks vs. Benefits of Medical Care,* Stanford professor Dr. Eugene Robin discusses how no one is keeping the real score on medical testing. He maintains that when the hidden costs are added up much of medical testing may not be such a good deal after all. Every medical test you undergo can give erroneous results that may lead to further unnecessary testing, a false diagnosis, or the wrong treatment—which could create extra risk rather than benefit. Despite the appearance of precision, most medical tests are far from perfect.

This chapter will furnish you with facts about some of the more "popular" medical tests, as well as emphasize and reemphasize the following guideline to medical testing. If the outcome of a medical test or procedure is not going to change your treatment, don't have it done.

Danger on the Treadmill

Avid runner and sportswriter Dan Levin described in *Sports Illustrated* (May 20, 1985) his own nightmarish odyssey that began one day as he was running through New York City's Central Park. In the middle of his daily six-mile run, a jolt of pain hit him in the chest. Thinking he had experienced "It," Levin got help immediately. Although his chest pain quickly disappeared, it was replaced by a lengthy and frustrating search for an answer to his problem. Several months later, after many sleepless nights and $8,983 worth of medical bills for seven different heart tests—including one that has killed a few people—he was told that his coronary arteries were normal and that his chest pain had almost certainly been of musculoskeletal origin. It was the result of overexercising and had nothing whatsoever to do with heart disease. Unfortunately Dan Levin's story has become an increasingly familiar one: people going through batteries of medical testing without good reason and suffering not-so-minor negative consequences.

Exercise stress testing: do the benefits outweigh the disadvantages? Let's look at the facts.

This costly examination is widely performed, allegedly to clarify the nature of unexplained chest pain and as a preventative screening procedure in executive medical examinations. It's a money-maker for hospitals and cardiologists, but its appropriateness is questionable in many cases, as Henry Soloman discusses in his book *The Exercise Myth*. To begin with, the test adds very little to a clinical interview. If your physician, in taking your clinical history, finds evidence of heart disease, the chances are about 90 percent that you do have coronary artery disease. A positive exercise test will only raise the odds to about 98 percent, which really would not change your situation very much. Either way, you most likely have heart disease.

Now consider the other possibilities. If you have no symptoms suggestive of heart disease, your probability of *not having* the disease is roughly 95 percent. How much more will you know if you undergo an exercise stress test? If the test is positive, in the absence of a suggestive history, the odds are still 75 percent in your favor of *not* having heart disease. And if you are a woman, the results of the tests are even more meaningless. A positive exercise stress test in a young woman without symptoms suggestive of heart disease is downright reassuring: the results will be *wrong* 80 percent of the time!

So you do not have a lot to gain from exercise stress testing, while you do have something to lose. First of all, the test itself is not without danger. Fatalities do occur, albeit rarely. Second, as we have seen, the results are often erroneous. Between 5 percent and 35 percent of individuals who take this test have false results suggestive of heart disease; and in certain groups, such as women with minor heart valve abnormalities, the false positive rate is considerably higher.

In the March 15, 1989, issue of the *Annals of Internal Medicine*, Stanford University researchers reported the results of an extensive cost-benefit analysis of exercise stress testing. They summarized their results this way: "The model predicts that screening would increase the life expectancy of sixty-year-old men at average risk by at most twelve days. Sixty-year-old men with no risk factors for coronary artery disease would derive less benefit, as would women and younger men." Not the kind of results that would encourage you to go right out and get tested.

In any form of medical testing, a false test result is usually just the beginning of your problems. Understandably there will be pressure from your physician to get to the bottom of this by your undergoing additional studies. With respect to heart disease, if coronary angiography is the next stop on the testing circuit, the level of danger has jumped significantly. Coronary angiography involves injecting a dye visible on X-ray into a person's coronary arteries and looking for narrowing. This procedure sometimes leads to coronary arterial spasm, which cuts off flow to the heart and causes a heart attack. Herein lies the greatest danger of unnecessary medical tests. Spurious results lead to more testing with potential complications, sometimes even death.

Consider a second test, "pulmonary wedge pressure." Although this one is not nearly as well known to the public, it has been widely used in the diagnosis and management of people who have suffered heart attacks. Of the 1.5 million annual heart attack victims, about 300,000 never make it to the hospital alive. Those who do meet up with an onslaught of modern medical technology, including continuous electronic monitoring, a barrage of medications, and extensive medical testing. One of the tests involves passing a thin-bore plastic catheter through a peripheral vein and threading it up through the pulmonary artery, the major artery to the lung. At the tip of the catheter is a pressure sensor that allows the patient's doctor to follow the pulmonary blood pressure and flow. This measure had been considered an important indicator of heart functioning.

In October 1987, based on a review of 3,263 records from sixteen hospitals, researchers from the University of Massachusetts Medical School reported a disturbing finding. Heart attack victims who had been catheterized were *twice* as likely to die as those who had not had the procedure. This was true even when the researchers had controlled for the severity of the heart attack. The procedure also was found to provide no advantage to patients who survived their heart attack and returned home. They fared no better in terms of long-term survival than did those patients who had not had the test.

Many medical tests are far from innocuous procedures; there should be a good reason for undergoing them. It's in your interest to make sure that that's the case.

Diseases Created by Tests

Sometimes medical tests create new diseases. Hypoglycemia is a case in point. Over the past decade many books have been written about this condition. A vast array of symptoms including fatigue, anxiety, personality disorders, sexual dysfunction, and mental dullness have been attributed to low blood sugar. Refined sugar, like salt, has become a notorious villain of our times.

The lore about sugar was greatly abetted by the widespread use of the oral glucose tolerance test. The person being tested has his blood sugar measured and then is given a bottle of highly concentrated sugary liquid. At various intervals for several hours, the person's blood sugar is retested. The idea is that normal people show a steep rise in blood sugar the first hour, but by two hours, it is back to normal due to the action of the body's own insulin. If not, something is wrong. The person could be showing early signs of diabetes or could have a condition known as "reactive hypoglycemia." On the basis of this test thousands of people have been falsely diagnosed and unnecessarily treated.

The "disease" was the product of the test itself, according to an article in *Data Centrum* (September/October 1985). The sugar "loading" was far in excess of what would be normally encountered in daily living. The people were reacting "abnormally" only in response to an abnormally huge slug of sugar. Today it is recommended that symptoms of low blood sugar be evaluated with a more realistic mixed meal of 50 percent carbohydrate, 35 percent fat, and 15 percent protein. When this standard is used, reactive hypoglycemia rarely turns up.

Not long ago a friend of mine called me about his older daughter. She had gone to see a physician for a routine examination only to leave his office in tears. She'd been told she suffered from "mitral valve prolapse." It sounded bad. Understandably my friend was concerned. He wanted to know how serious it was. I was happy to reassure him that more than likely his daughter was suffering from a *test-created* disease that would be of little consequence.

The vast majority of people who are given this diagnosis, mainly young women, have nothing to worry about. Mitral valve prolapse is a diagnosis that's currently in style. You complain of vague symptoms such as fatigue and anxiety, your doctor listens to your chest, and the mystery is solved. A faint clicking sound gives the case away. You have mitral valve prolapse. To verify this, the physician sends you for special ultrasound imaging of your heart called "echocardiography." Sure enough, the picture shows slight bulging of the mitral valve. Case closed. Except that now you have to live with the diagnosis of heart disease.

According to a report in the *New England Journal of Medicine* in 1985, studies have shown that most individuals with mitral valve prolapse do not have serious heart disease. The condition seems to be a normal variant, the reflection of a highly sensitive test rather than the sign of real heart pathology. Although a version of this syndrome in older men can pose serious problems, the vast majority of young women in this country who are diagnosed as having mitral valve prolapse, like my friend's daughter, can rest easy. They are victims of a phantom disease.

Incidentally, relieved by what I told him, my friend chuckled and related to me how thirty-five years before he had been discharged from the service for a "heart problem." The doctor had apparently heard a click of some sort and thought he was a bad risk. Once out of the service my friend went on to become a highly successful lawyer. At age sixty-two, he has yet to suffer from his "heart problem."

Ronald Reagan's Disease

When the president of the United States gets cancer, people pay attention. The discovery that Ronald Reagan had colon cancer brought a quick public response. In a survey of Chicago households, 62 percent of the respondents, up 15 percent from two years earlier, said they would ask for a stool blood test at their next doctor's visit. While it's commendable that more people are knowledgeable about colon cancer—the second most common killing cancer—the screening test for it is not without its problems.

The test for colon cancer actually is not a cancer test at all. It's a test for blood in the stool. Individuals younger than forty-five years old have little reason to consider the test, since colon cancer rarely strikes before that age. Furthermore, more than 50 percent of patients eventually discovered to have colon cancer *do not* have a positive stool blood test, according to an article in *The Medical Letter* (January 17, 1986). In these cases the test creates a false sense of security.

Of those people with a positive test, *90 percent will not* have colon cancer. Positive results are most often due to blood from hemorrhoids, ulcers, or gastric bleeding caused by substances such as aspirin and alcohol. Like most medical screening tests, the tests for colon cancer should always be repeated before putting too much stock in the results. Otherwise you run the risk of being subjected to more invasive procedures on the basis of a false test.

Don't get me wrong: I am not arguing against having this test done. For people aged forty and over—especially those who have a family history of this cancer—it's a worthwhile test, and the costs are minimal. With self-testing kits now available, you can even conduct this test in the privacy of your own home. As with any medical test, however, you need to keep the limitations of self-testing for colon cancer in mind. If the test is positive, it is always a good idea to repeat it. If it is still positive, consult your doctor.

I have an additional caveat for people fifty years and older. In this age group, this test should not be used as a substitute for sigmoidoscopy. The blood test is not sensitive enough for people entering that period in their lives when the risk of colon cancer rises sharply. After age fifty, sigmoidoscopy should be done every few years. Reports from the front indicate that it is not as bad as you might imagine. Patients report that they experience far less discomfort from sigmoidoscopy (performed with a *flexible* sigmoidoscope) than they had anticipated.

The Limits of Testing

Medical tests are only as good as the machines or technicians that carry them out. The Pap smear is a good sample. A scraping of cells taken from a woman's cervix is smeared onto a glass slide. A trained technician examines the slide under a microscope, looking for early cellular changes that foreshadow cervical cancer. When these changes are detected, preventive steps can be taken before cervical cancer has a chance to develop. The idea behind it is excellent. Physicians and their female patients have come to put great trust in the Pap smear, making it one of the most common laboratory tests in America.

Unfortunately, this trust is not completely deserved. The Pap smear turns out to be one of the more inaccurate medical tests being commonly performed today. As it is presently done in many laboratories across the country, the Pap smear fails to identify roughly one out of every four cases of cervical cancer or its precursor (dysplasia). The problem is human error.

The Pap smear test cannot be automated. Each slide must be read by a trained technician. In a chilling investigative report, November 2, 1987, the *Wall Street Journal* described Pap smear analysis in "Pap factories" or "mills" where technicians may read four times as many specimens per year as medical experts recommend. Some of these technicians work two or more jobs, receiving as little as forty-five cents to perform the key analysis on a test that may cost thirty-five dollars or more. In some instances laboratories let technicians take the slides home to screen. (The idea of a slide possibly being read on the kitchen table next to a jar of peanut butter does not inspire a lot of confidence.) These "Pap mills" survive by underbidding more reputable laboratories.

The point is that the Pap smear can only be trusted when it is performed in competent and reliable laboratories. The message for a woman is this: Ask your doctor about the laboratory he uses. Is it accredited? What is the workload level? Pap smears in the wrong hands cannot be trusted.

Consider now a different kind of test, as many people are currently asking themselves the question, "Should I be tested for AIDS?" In part the answer depends on whether or not the person understands and is willing to accept the limitations of the test. For starters it is an *indirect* test. The so-called "AIDS Test" does not test for AIDS, or for that matter, even for the HIV virus thought to cause the disease. Rather it tests for antibodies that are produced when a person has been infected by the HIV virus. People who test positive are presumed to carry the virus and be capable of spreading it through intimate sexual contact or blood exchange.

The information we can get from the HIV antibody test is limited. It can tell us only a person's antibody status *at the time the test is done*. On the average it takes two to three months—in some cases several years or longer—for an infection to result in a positive test, so a negative result today may simply mean that the HIV infection is too recent to have shown up. Another limitation, often glossed over by those who call for universal mandatory AIDS testing as a way of bringing the epidemic under control, is that one-time testing indicates nothing about the future. Even if a person is truly negative today, this is no guarantee that he or she will be negative a year from now. The only way to obtain accurate information is to require that the test be repeated periodically in individuals who have had any risk of exposure since the last test. The logistical problems involved in repeatedly testing the entire population of the United States are truly mind-boggling.

Finally, although the two-test regimen for HIV antibodies is highly accurate, this does not eliminate the problem of "false positives" and "false negatives." Individuals at low risk for AIDS exposure run the risk of having a false positive test result. These people will be told that they are positive for HIV antibodies because the test is in error, not because of actual exposure. The *Journal of the American Medical Association* in 1987 projected that, if all couples getting married in the United States submitted to mandatory AIDS testing over a period of one year, there would be 350 individuals falsely determined to be positive.

For low-risk individuals deciding whether or not to have the AIDS test, there are several considerations. Currently, with the estimated prevalence of the AIDS virus in the general population at one per one thousand to one per ten thousand, the odds are very much in your favor that you would test negative. If you should decide to take the test and *should* test positive, there is a possibility that it's a false positive. The first thing you should do is make certain there has been a confirmatory test, and, if not, then have it done. If the test is still positive, have the two-step testing procedure repeated.

For persons who are high-risk for HIV exposure, given recent developments in the monitoring and early treatment of HIV infection, early testing is to be recommended. The potential benefits of having the infection closely monitored and treated if indicated outweigh the risks of erroneous testing.

Consider a more common type of test now: breast self-examination. Roughly 125,000 women each year develop breast cancer. For decades breast self-examination has been espoused as a way to detect breast cancer early. A 1987 report in the *Journal of the American Medical Association* has now raised serious questions about this form of testing. The United States Preventive Task Force reported that when compared with two well-proven methods for detecting breast cancer, breast self-examination was only 20 to 30 percent as sensitive.

The task force felt that reliance on self-examination ran the risk of drawing attention away from medical examinations (by health professionals skilled in finding breast lumps) and mammographies. When a special ranking system developed by the task force for rating preventive health services was used, breast self-examination got a "C" while the combination of mammography and medical examination got an "A."

So while breast self-examination may be simple, cheap, and safe, it has its limitations. When put to the test, it is not nearly as sensitive as two readily available alternatives. If a woman examines her own breasts, it should not be done as a substitute for these other measures. While in the past the radiation exposure from mammography was great enough to raise serious questions about the overall benefit, modern equipment exposes women to extremely small doses of radiation. (A woman undergoing mammography should make sure that modern equipment is being used.)

Sometimes a test tells us more than we need to know. As a result of the relatively low cost of automated blood testing, doctors often find themselves ordering more blood work than is indicated simply because the one test they are interested in is cheaper if performed as part of a larger package. It would appear to be a good deal for the patient: pay for one test, get ten free. But that is not always true. When the results of a panel of tests come back, there is a statistical likelihood that one out of the batch will be "abnormal." Now the physician is stuck. If nothing else, he or she has to follow up this "abnormal" result for medical-legal reasons. So, the results of one of the free tests (that were not indicated in the first place) give rise to more testing—and, more often than not, to unwarranted concern on the patient's part.

Similarly, sometimes greater test sensitivity results in the availability of more information than we might need or want. This has happened with some of the newer monoclonal pregnancy tests. The "diagnosis" of pregnancy now can be made even before the first day of the first missed period. The trade-off for being able to tell women a few days earlier whether or not they are pregnant is that now many more women will be made aware of miscarriages. A large percentage of all conceptions—one-third to one-half—abort spontaneously within nine to fourteen days of a missed period. In the past these were silent; now, thanks to the advances in pregnancy testing, they will be identified and cause anguish that women previously were spared.

The Basic Question

Despite the wonders of modern medical technology and the emphasis on sophisticated medical screening, medical tests are simply not always advisable. Remember that basic question you should always ask: Will the outcome have important bearing on my treatment? It is surprising how often tests are undertaken even when the answer to this question is negative.

Dr. David Sobel, co-author of *The People's Book of Medical Tests*, in an interview in *Health Action* (October 1985), describes a man who injured his knee in a skiing accident and was taken to an orthopedist. The physician recommended arthroscopy, a procedure in which a thin tube is inserted into the knee to visualize the damage and carry out treatment. The cost ranges between $500 and $1,000.

When the man asked what the procedure would show, the doctor responded, "A torn ligament, if you have one." And what would the treatment be if he did turn out to have a torn ligament? "You'll do knee rehabilitation exercises, and we'll see how it goes," came the reply. The man thought for a moment and then asked: "One last question. If I don't have an arthroscopy, what will the treatment be?" The doctor repeated himself somewhat sheepishly, "You'll do knee rehabilitation exercises and we'll see how it goes." Dr. Sobel reveals that the patient in the story was himself. Needless to say he passed up the arthroscopy, saving himself money, discomfort, and the unnecessary risk of joint infection or bleeding. He followed the important rule: *If the outcome of a medical test or procedure is not going to change your treatment, don't have it done.*

Today medical tests sometimes add up to about half the charges on a hospital bill. When tests are available, they are often given whether indicated or not, "just to be on the safe side." Doctors and consumers alike have become enamored of testing—the more the better. But many health tests, as we have seen, carry invisible risks. To undergo a medical test simply because it is available is not a sound reason for taking on those invisible risks.

Recently there has been a surge in consumer self-test kits coming on the market. Osco, a major drugstore chain, is experimenting with in-store medical testing booths. Customers can walk up to a shopping center kiosk and have any one of a number of medical tests performed. Some test results are available immediately; others can be picked up later or mailed to customers within forty-eight hours. The direction is clear. Medical testing will become more accessible. This will be viewed by consumer activists as a long-overdue development. And well it may be, but the dangers of indiscriminate testing apply as much to self-testing as to any other form of health testing. When it comes to medical tests, more is not necessarily better.

Points to Remember

1. When you have a medical test, three outcomes are possible— a correct result, a false positive, or a false negative. Two of them are bad news! Make sure you need a medical test before you have it.

2. If you are tempted to undergo exercise stress testing, don't— until a cardiologist has convinced you beyond doubt that the potential benefit outweighs the risks.

3. There's a new kind of disease. It's called *Excessive Medical Testing*. The best treatment is prevention.

4. The first thing to do when you obtain an abnormal result on a medical test is to have it repeated. Accept no less. (The only exceptions would be tests that carry significant risk.)

5. If the outcome of a medical test or procedure is not going to change your treatment, don't agree to it.

▸ ▸ ▸ ▸ ▸

In the space of one hundred and seventy-six years the lower Mississippi has shortened itself two hundred miles. That is an average of a trifle over one mile and a third per year. Therefore, any calm person, who is not blind or idiotic, can see that in the Old Oölitic Silurian Period, just a million years ago next November, the Lower Mississippi River was upward of one million three hundred thousand miles long and stuck out over the Gulf of Mexico like a fishing rod. . . .

There is something fascinating about science. One gets such wholesale returns of conjecture out of such a trifling investment of fact.

—Mark Twain, *Life on the Mississippi*

CHAPTER SEVEN

▸ ▸ ▸ ▸ ▸ ▸ ▸ ▸ ▸

Statistical Games Health Hype Plays

For most of us, statistics holds no great fascination. It's pretty dull stuff. In the right hands, though, statistics is a valuable analytic tool. It has the power to reveal important distinctions that otherwise would go unnoticed. That's why in a wide range of fields from insurance to medical research, statistics has become indispensable.

But statistics has a dual personality. As Mark Twain pointed out long ago, statistics can be used to hide the truth equally as well as illuminating it. "There are three kinds of lies," he claimed. "Lies, damn lies, and statistics." Whether by design or not, statistics misleads us as much as it informs us.

There are three favorite statistical games that health fiction uses to its advantage: Risk Rook, Molehill Madness, and Everybody's Got It. In this chapter, you'll learn some things you need to know in order to see through statistical games.

Risk Rook

Risk Rook is played by pointing out a player's risk—any risk—and then maneuvering so as to make the player feel the risk is so great that it may endanger his life. Health hype wins the game when the player becomes desperate. The key maneuver in Risk Rook is a statistical ploy known as "relative risk."

Relative risk is a journalist's (and medical researcher's) dream. It's a catchy kind of shorthand that gives the appearance of neatly summarizing health risk studies. You may not recognize it by its official name; but undoubtedly you've run across it.

Typically, relative risk is stated like this: Your chances of getting a certain disease are so many times greater because you do this or you don't do that. For example, if you are a middle-aged man with the three major risk factors, your chances of getting coronary heart disease are increased eightfold. That is, your relative risk is eight times greater than another man your age and health status who doesn't have these risk factors. If you are a woman who uses tampons, your relative risk of developing toxic shock syndrome is sixteen times greater than a woman who doesn't use tampons. Oral contraceptive users run a risk ten times greater than nonusers of developing thromboembolism, a serious and sometimes life-threatening condition that results when clots (usually from veins deep in the leg) break off and lodge elsewhere in the body, such as in the lungs. Heavy smokers contract lung cancer twenty times more frequently than nonsmokers.

All of these statements are true, as far as they go. It's just that they don't go far enough. They leave out half the story—the most important half, I might add.

Relative risk has become a universal language for translating medical research findings. And why not? It's such a simple way of letting people know where they stand. Only one thing is wrong: relative risk has an impish and obsessive habit of overstating the case. This is why it's one of health fiction's favorite tools.

Let's look at what it does in presenting the risk of an older woman having a Down's Syndrome child.

Couples who delay having children may find themselves confronted with scary predictions about Down's Syndrome. Stated as a relative risk, the situation does indeed sound ominous. Compared to a twenty-five-year-old woman, a woman aged forty has approximately a ten-times-greater chance of having a Down's Syndrome baby, making the risk appear absolutely horrendous (at least until one looks at the actual figures).

For a twenty-five-year-old woman, the incidence of a Down's Syndrome baby is roughly 1 out of every 1,200 live births. At age forty—despite a much greater relative risk—the occurrence is only 10 out of every 1,200. Stated another way, out of every 1,200 live babies born to forty-year-old women, 1,190 will *not have* Down's Syndrome. Although the odds at age forty are not as favorable as one might like, they are not nearly as bleak as relative risk would have us believe.

For another example we have only to turn to the Great California Milk Debate. It well illustrates relative risk's almost unlimited capacity for blowing things out of proportion. It began when California health officials put raw milk drinkers on notice. The story broke in the *Los Angeles Times* on March 31, 1984, with the scare headline, "Raw-Milk Drinkers Reported More at Risk Than Smokers." They then announced that the threat of contracting *Salmonella dublin*, a potentially lethal bacterium, was *158 times greater* for drinkers of raw milk than for pasteurized-milk drinkers. Health authorities from around the country expressed grave concern over the dangers of raw milk. Dr. Mark J. Finch, medical epidemiologist for the Centers for Disease Control in Atlanta, commented: "A risk factor of 158 is extremely high. I can't think of any relative risk factors that are higher." The finding was described as "spectacular" by Dr. Richard J. Brand of the University of California, Berkeley, School of Public Health, who concluded: "We have a noteworthy health problem here and people should be alerted to the risks of drinking raw milk."

It was sounding bad for the raw-milk drinkers of California. But in part, this was because only one side of the story had been told. The officials had been extremely careful not to state the *actual* risk involved in drinking raw milk. Of those people who do not drink raw milk, three out of every one million contract *Salmonella dublin*. (The odds are slightly more than being struck by lightning.) A risk, yes, but in the overall scheme of things nothing to be overly concerned about. Given this small baseline risk, raw-milk drinkers—despite their 158-times-greater risk—are looking at odds of five out of every ten thousand! Not the kind of risk to panic over.

Relative risk is a statistical magnifying glass. It transforms minor threats into major dangers. Unfortunately, when research is translated into newspaper or magazine columns or into sixty seconds of radio or television coverage, relative risk may be the only thing that is left. Health news becomes Risk Rook.

In the mid-1980s there was a surge of concern about teenage suicide. Major magazines and newspapers carried articles about the tragic epidemic sweeping our country. Legislatures awarded large research grants to get to the bottom of this scourge and develop ways of preventing it. Several films for television were made depicting the pain and agony of teenagers struggling with the thought of taking their own lives and of the pain experienced by the surviving family and loved ones. Massive discussion groups were held in schools to get this potential killer out in the open.

Almost as suddenly as this explosive issue of teenage suicide burst upon the scene, it faded away. What was this all about?

As tragic as it is, teenage suicide is relatively rare. Even during this period of great national concern, it remained an infrequent event. But statements about the relative risk of teenage suicide made it appear far more common that it was. It was stated that suicide among fifteen- to twenty-four-year-olds had become the second leading cause of death and was three times higher than in 1960. Stated in this fashion, teenage suicide appeared to be a raging epidemic. Nothing could have been further from the truth.

Mostly, it was a play on numbers. The actual rate of suicide among teenagers in 1960 was 4 to 5 per 100,000. By 1980, after the rate had *tripled*, still, it was only 12 to 13 per 100,000. While it was true that suicide was the second-leading cause of death among teenagers, what went unsaid was that teenagers do not have high death rates—even the *leading* causes of death do not occur all that frequently. Also, seldom made was the point that the leading cause of death—automobile accidents—was far more frequent than the number-two cause, suicide.

The loss of even one teenager to suicide is a terrible human tragedy. But nothing is gained by portraying the problem as epidemic. It well illustrates the power of relative risk to mislead us.

Whereas a research scientist may find an intriguing hypothesis in the fact that one person has a risk several times greater than another, for consumers this is not such an important point. You want to know what your actual odds are. Rather than helping, statements of relative risk can mislead you. The next time you come across a story about a new health risk, look for the actual numbers. Keep in mind, when it says your risk is four times as great, it could be that your odds are four out of ten or four out of a million! *You can't tell unless you have the rest of the story: How likely are individuals who are not at greater risk to have the problem?* Only when you know this can you understand what a risk of four times as great really means.

Keeping health risks in perspective is tricky business.

Molehill Madness

Health hype's second statistical game is Molehill Madness. It starts with the selection of a medical finding of little consequence. The object is to transform a minor finding into a dramatic health news headline. Health hype wins when a majority of consumers are convinced of a major medical breakthrough. The key strategy in Molehill Madness is a play on the word "significant."

In everyday usage, when we say something is "significant," we mean important, out of the ordinary. It would be highly irregular, to say the least, to routinely describe matters of minor consequence as "highly significant." But in medical research, things are different. What is "significant" statistically actually can be quite unimportant. In fact, in medical research trivial findings are routinely described as "highly significant." In his book *Interpreting the Medical Literature*, Stephen Gehlbach discusses this paradox, which arises because "significance" doesn't refer to the importance of a finding, but rather to whether or not the finding has occurred by chance. If it's a chance outcome, it is dubbed "insignificant." If, on the other hand, the finding is a consequence of the variable under study, it is declared "significant" or even "highly significant." The less likely that it occurred by chance, the more "significant" it is. *Importance* is not a consideration until health hype steps in.

When the word "significance" is picked up in the popular media, its unorthodox meaning is not explained. "New Medical Findings Highly Significant" makes good copy, but it probably does not mean what readers think it means.

Medical researchers try to design their studies so that they can trust the results. They don't want to be left wondering if the findings are only a product of chance. They have done this by working out a standard known as a "p-value." (Stay with me here, this gets a little dense.) Typically, the accepted p-value for medical research is expressed as .05 or less. This means that if the outcome of the study is such that it could have been expected to occur *purely by chance less than 5 percent of the time*, it is a "significant" finding. In contrast, if the outcome would have occurred by chance *more than 5 percent of the time*, it is "insignificant." The nature of the results matters not a whit. "Significant" means that whatever the outcome is—monumental or trivial (a cure for cancer or eye twitches in spotted lizards)—it was not a chance finding, 95 percent sure. This is why trivial medical research findings truthfully can be labeled "significant." *Insignificant significance*. It's a confusing concept.

Robert Sapolsky, a Stanford professor, wrote a charming piece about insignificant significance entitled "The Case of the Falling Nightwatchmen" in *Discover* magazine (July 1987). He put the matter slightly differently: for him there are strong facts and weak facts. Science certifies both kinds as "significant." But in the common sense use of the term, of course, they are not the same. Scientific truths are not all equal. The best thing to do with some of them is to ignore them.

Sapolsky illustrates his point by contrasting the two kinds of facts. The deadly organism anthrax will kill most people within forty-eight hours if it is not treated with antibiotics. But if treated immediately, almost 100 percent of people infected survive. That's a strong fact! Contrast this to the moon's influence on nightwatchmen. As the lunar cycle progresses, the moon exerts a changing gravitational influence. "If nightwatchmen of equal weight and density tumble from the top of a building each midnight, the force with which they hit the ground will be influenced by the distance of the moon from the earth that night." In other words, there is a tiny change in the force with which a falling nightwatchman would strike the ground depending on where the moon is positioned. A scientific fact? Yes. Of any practical consequence? No. It's a weak fact, an example of insignificant significance.

Several years ago a famous study, known as the Stanford Heart Disease Prevention Program, was conducted in a three-county area in California. Through a long-term program of community health education, Stanford researchers attempted to reduce the major risk factors associated with heart disease. Subsequently, they reported "significant results" that received international acclaim as evidence for the potential of health education in reducing heart disease. But what were the actual results?

Let's focus on smoking behavior. The outcome was described as a *significant* decrease in smoking. After two years, smokers in the experimental group had reduced their smoking to twenty cigarettes a day. How far had they come? Not very far. At the start they were smoking twenty-two cigarettes. That's a net reduction of two cigarettes a day. The practical significance of this is questionable.

Inconsequential medical findings often pass statistical standards. Keep in mind that *statistical* significance is a traditional requirement for publication of medical research while *practical* importance is not.

One of my favorite examples of insignificant significance comes from a study I recall reading several years ago. The investigator randomly selected one hundred people with high blood pressure and one hundred who were free of this problem. The two groups were then compared on a long list of factors. In medical research this is what is known as a "fishing expedition." Unsure as to what exactly he was looking for, the researcher threw in a lot of things hoping to find at least a few that would distinguish individuals with high blood pressure from those without it. Of the one hundred factors studied, two were statistically significant.

First, individuals with high blood pressure had more letters in their last name. Second, they were much more likely to be born during the first three and a half days of the week. So, the researcher dutifully reported a "significant" association between longer last names and birthdays during the first half of the week and high blood pressure! As far as I know the outcome of this study was not picked up by the wire services or by network television, but the same cannot be said for many studies not all that dissimilar from this one.

Large-scale medical studies command great media attention. The belief seems to be that if a massive number of people have been studied, the results are more likely to be true. What's overlooked, however, is this: the larger a study sample size, the *smaller the differences required to achieve statistical significance*. A few years ago a Frenchman named Michel Gauquelin compared the astrological signs of several million people with various lines of work. He found a highly "significant" difference between military people and artists. They had different signs—much more so than would be predicted by chance. Fascinating, until one realizes that in studies of this size, tiny differences become "significant." On the one hand, we can feel confident that the differences actually exist. On the other, they may well be so small as not to be of any consequence except to statisticians.

Statistical significance has yet another troubling aspect. Alfred Berg, writing in the *Journal of Family Practice*, found that at least five out of every one hundred medical studies showing "significant results" are actually erroneous. Given that thousands of medical studies are reported each year, a 5 percent rate of error means a whopping number of false reports. And this is when statistical analyses are correctly applied. To make matters worse, medical researchers often do not apply statistical methods properly. In 1978, the *New England Journal of Medicine* reported a survey of seventy-one studies reported as *insignificant*. In a majority of these studies, the researchers were wrong. Their results were actually "significant"!

Statistical techniques are fallible. And there's usually a world of difference between statistical and actual significance. The next time you come across a headline proclaiming "significant results," read the small print; make sure it's not just another case of health hype putting insignificant significance to work by making mountains out of molehills.

Everybody's Got It

Think back to the story of Chicken Little. Hit on the head by a falling acorn, Chicken Little assumes that the sky is falling and that everywhere everybody is in danger. Everybody's Got It is a game based on Chicken Little's logic. Health hype latches on to the findings from a medical study of persons X, Y, and Z. Then while persons A, B, and C are not watching, the results from persons X, Y, and Z are slipped into the envelopes of A, B, and C. If they don't notice the difference and if they accept the findings in their envelopes as their own, health hype wins the game. Overgeneralizing is the game's basic move.

Researchers—as well as the media—routinely overgeneralize. They are not content to stick to their findings, and there's a simple reason for this. When seen for what they are, most research findings are quite limited in their application.

For example, if laboratory rats are fed astronomical amounts of artificial sweetener and subsequently develop bladder cancer, the only thing that can be concluded scientifically is that rats who eat loads of artificial sweetener are at higher risk for getting bladder cancer. It's not difficult to see that such a finding would not create a lot of excitement. So the temptation is to fudge a little; to speculate beyond the study itself. Urged on by the media, medical researchers overgeneralize their conclusions. In this instance facts about rats become speculations masquerading as scientific findings about humans.

Overgeneralizing is not limited to applying animal studies to humans. Most medical studies on humans cannot be applied on a broad scale. For example, the effects of a medication on a group of elderly women can't be automatically extended to teenagers. And even when the research subjects are more representative of the general population, generalizations are difficult to make. Why? Because a study of a few cases simply cannot be trusted when applied to everyone. Despite human similarities, individual differences are great. This seriously limits the conclusions that can be drawn from any study for the rest of us.

For the purpose of illustration, consider overgeneralization in a different context. For years certain automobile insurance companies engaged in a practice known as "redlining." Based on a history of regional automobile insurance claims, the company set its insurance rates depending on *where* a person lived. A certain percentage profit was added to the calculated premium and, presto, the company had a no-fail, sure-profit system. Good for the company but bad for the safe-driving consumer who happened to live in a high-rated area. Regardless of driving record, if the person lived in the "wrong part of town," the premium would be excessive, equal to that charged to high-risk drivers. Under this system, good drivers paid more and bad drivers less than they would if judged individually. It mattered little to the insurance companies, because in the end the figures all balanced out and a profit was made.

Suggesting that everyone should become obsessively concerned with heart disease because it is the overall number-one killer is akin to redlining. This simply does not follow. Only certain individuals (because of a strong family history or notable indicators of suscepti-bility to heart disease) should be *very* concerned. For starters heart disease, particularly premature heart disease, is largely a male prob-lem. On the average, women have far less risk for this disease than men. Their chances of coming down with heart disease are comparatively low.

In the Health Hype Hall of Fame we reviewed a study of middle-aged men with extremely high cholesterol levels treated with the cholesterol-lowering agent cholestyramine. When the researchers concluded that *all* Americans over the age of two should adopt a low-cholesterol diet, they were committing a serious error of overgenera-lizing. This was not a study of women or children or even men with normal cholesterol levels, and it had absolutely nothing to do with a low-cholesterol diet.

Much of medical research is conducted on people who already suffer from certain diseases or who, for one reason or another, are at considerable risk. "Caution" should be the watchword when applying these findings to the average person. Unfortunately, it is not. After all, you don't get the reader's or viewer's attention by giving all the reasons why what you are about to say probably doesn't apply.

Assume for a moment you are one of thousands of Americans suffering from the heart pain known as angina pectoris, a condition arising from atherosclerotic narrowing of the coronary arteries. You hear of the growing ranks of people undergoing bypass surgery, now the most common operation in males over the age of fifty. You read articles describing the tremendous relief patients have experienced after this form of surgery. You begin to seriously consider it for yourself.

So far so good, but before you fully commit yourself to this course of action, you need to assure yourself that your situation resembles that of the patients who profit most from this operation. In other words, you need to individualize your decision as much as possible. One study you would definitely want to review is the Coronary Artery Surgery Study.

This was a study of 780 patients who were considered excellent candidates for bypass surgery. Most of them had moderate heart pain that was responsive to medication. All of them had at least one severely narrowed coronary artery. Half of the patients were simply continued on medication while the other half underwent a bypass operation. The outcome was unexpected.

After five years, patients receiving medication alone were doing just as well as those who had undergone the surgery. There was no difference in survival rate or the occurrence of heart attack, and the chances of returning to work were similar for the two groups. Although patients had some lessening of pain following surgery, the discomfort from the operation itself was considerable, not to mention the expense.

Based on this study—and you would want to consider others as well—as long as your coronary artery disease responds to medication and is not progressing, surgery is probably not a wise choice. If in the future your condition changes, you can always reconsider. To plunge ahead now, joining the push for bypass surgery, would be falling victim to overgeneralization.

Survey research is a specialized field. You and I know it best because of the political polls and opinion surveys that we read about. Critical to this kind of research is the creation of a representative sample. If the findings are going to be valid, then the people who are sampled must reflect the larger population. Often these surveys are conducted on less than two thousand individuals. The number is not nearly as critical as is ensuring that the people selected are representative.

In 1987 a book entitled *Women and Love: A Cultural Revolution in Progress*, by Shere Hite, was published. Had Ms. Hite written the book as an expression of her own personal opinions derived from personal interviews, there would have been no problem. Instead, the book was promoted as a scientific study of how American women view men and love relationships.

Putting together a representative account of American women's attitudes about men and love is quite an undertaking. The first and most crucial step would be to secure a representative sample. It was at this initial juncture that Ms. Hite hit a major stumbling block. After mailing out 100,000 questionnaires, she received back only 4,500 (4.5 percent). One reviewer described this return rate as "what you would pray for if you were in the junk mail business." Given this poor response, any serious researcher would have had no choice but to either start over or "consider another line of business." In fact a response rate of less than 50 percent generally disqualifies survey studies from being reported in respectable journals. But this did not stop Shere Hite.

She took the information and wrote her report as though the samples were representative of American women. Journalists and radio and television commentators across the country then compounded the problem by reporting it as an important scientific study showing that modern American women were bitterly fed up with men. The cover of *Time* magazine asked the question: "Are Women Fed Up?" Inside, the findings were discussed in an article entitled, "Back Off, Buddy."

"Scientific" is not an appropriate characterization of Hite's study. Pseudoscience would be more like it, or—as Carol Tavris, psychologist and writer, described it in a *Los Angeles Times* article—"social science-fiction." This is not to say that Ms. Hite is necessarily incorrect in her conclusions, but if she's right, it's not on the basis of valid research. Her results contrast sharply with those obtained from far more representative samples. Hite found that 88 percent of women said the men in their lives avoided talking things over. An ABC/

Washington Post telephone poll conducted shortly after publication of Hite's book reported 33 percent. Hite racked up headlines across the country with her claim that "70 percent of women married more than five years are having sex outside of marriage." A representative survey in *Redbook* found 29 percent.

Women and Love is actually based on a very narrow perspective. The sources were women in therapy, fans of Hite's previous books, or group joiners. They were by no means representative of American women. From the views they expressed, they appear to have been a rather unhappy lot, angry and resentful of men.

The Hite report is a splendid example of overgeneralization. And of all the statistical games that health hype plays, overgeneralization is probably its favorite. That's what makes Everybody's Got It such a commonly encountered health fiction ploy.

Points to Remember

1. Relative risk is a statistical magnifying glass. It exaggerates health risk. What really matters are the actual odds.

2. Most statistical significance has little to do with the real world. Many "significant" medical findings are of trivial importance. Don't lose sleep over them. Remember: Insignificant significance!

3. Most medical findings apply only to some of us. Health hype seldom if ever mentions this. It's not good for sales!

4. Take Mark Twain's words to heart: "There are three kinds of lies. Lies, damn lies, and statistics." Some things never change.

5. And keep in mind: statistically you can prove that most Miami residents are born Cuban and die Jewish!

▸ ▸ ▸ ▸ ▸

I was eating a corned-beef sandwich as I read the
Surgeon General's report on the current state of the
American diet. . . .

What I was reading, unfortunately, told me in no
uncertain terms that the food which I was so happily
consuming was not what I should be eating if I wanted
to live forever. The corned-beef sandwich on rye,
topped with Russian dressing, cole slaw, and mustard,
which tasted so very good, was—in the eyes of the
government—a festering mass of excessive fat,
sodium, and cholesterol.

—Merrill Shindler, *Los Angeles Times*
August 4, 1988

▶ ▶ ▶ ▶ ▶ ▶ ▶ ▶ ▶

CHAPTER EIGHT

What Medical Studies Can't Tell You

Although medical science has made incredible technological advancements, it has definite limits. One of the most problematic, as we have seen, is its inability to individualize its findings. Since most of its conclusions are derived from studies of *groups* of individuals (who may differ considerably from you or I), medical science has a devil of a time precisely relating its findings to any given person. Instead, it often acts as though one-size-fits-all. Seldom is this the case.

A second drawback relates to the nonexperimental nature of most medical research involving humans; instead, correlational studies are used, drawing connections between one thing and another for its findings. These studies are seriously limited in what they tell us, for there is no way to prove that the connections they turn up have a cause-and-effect relationship.

Medical science has some of the answers, but not all. A healthy skepticism on your part could prove to be good for your health.

Appearances Don't Necessarily Make It So

From infancy on, we have a tendency to mistake correlation for cause and effect. If, while looking over at mother, we stumble and fall, we likely may attribute the accident to mother. As we get older, we become less prone to this mistake, but the tendency never goes away completely.

Many a medical myth owes its existence to this confusion. Consider the alleged medicinal value of leeches. In certain cultures leeches are considered a sign of health, because in those locales it's common knowledge that healthy people are often infested with leeches whereas sick people are not. The fact is leeches do not make people healthy. It's just that they can't tolerate the heat from the bodies of people ridden with fever. So they relinquish their attachment to feverish individuals in favor of those with normal temperatures—thus falsely earning their reputation as agents of health.

Ludicrous conclusions result when the distinction between cause and correlation is forgotten. For example, the incidence of AIDS has risen along with the sale of VCRs. Do VCRs cause AIDS? The number of registered prostitutes has paralleled the rise of automobile sales in Tokyo. Do automobile sales cause a rise in prostitution; or, perhaps the other way around, does prostitution lead to greater car sales? People who smoke are less likely to develop Parkinson's disease. Cause and effect? Unlikely. These relationships are correlational, arising if not from pure coincidence, then from their tie to another common factor.

Several years ago Dr. Lester Breslow (now professor and dean emeritus at the UCLA School of Public Health) directed a ten-year study of the health habits of seven thousand adults in Alameda County, California. He found seven simple practices associated with increased length of life: regular physical activity, no smoking, moderate or no use of alcohol, seven to eight hours of sleep each night, maintenance of proper weight, eating breakfast regularly, and avoiding eating between meals. Based on this study, a forty-five-year-old man who engaged in six or seven of these practices could expect to live eleven years longer than his counterpart who engaged in three or fewer practices.

Notice that nothing in this study *proves* that these seven factors actually cause people to live longer. They could be coincidental findings. Those people who lived longer might have something else special about them that the researchers did not even consider. The study simply could not prove this one way or the other. But when the popular press stumbled onto Dr. Breslow's findings, it was off to the races.

Around the world these seven practices were portrayed as the proven cause of longer life. As Dr. Breslow tells it, this study has now been "rediscovered" by the media on several occasions and each time presented as "new findings" showing how seven simple practices make you live longer.

Let's look at another example: Dr. Lee Salk, a nationally recognized authority on child care, and his associates made headlines when they reported on teen suicide a few years ago. But what they reported and what their study showed were two different things. They had studied 156 teenagers, 52 of whom eventually committed suicide before age twenty. Despite looking at forty-six different factors, Dr. Salk found that the teenagers who committed suicide were no different from those who did not, with one exception: they were three to four times more likely to have had health problems as infants. Now, you would think it would be fairly obvious that this does not prove that being sick as an infant *causes* teenage suicide. Dr. Salk missed the obvious, however. He reported his findings in the prestigious British medical journal *Lancet*, and the popular press played it big. "Birth Trauma: A Factor in Teen Suicide?" headlined *USA Today* (March 19, 1985), and the *San Francisco Examiner* (March 21, 1985) speculated: "Teen-age Suicides May Have Lost Fear of Dying at Birth."

Dr. Salk himself, while quick to point out that his study did not establish cause and effect, fell into speculating as though it did. "Conceivably," he said, "experiencing near-death has some physiological effect on the individual that weakens their fear of death. In later stressful life experiences, they may be more inclined to end their lives as a means of coping." He likened these infants to "runt" pups rejected instinctively by mother dogs "to enhance the strength of the species [and] not to pass weaknesses into the species' genetic pool."

We are talking here about a single study that found a statistical association between health problems around the time of birth and subsequent suicide as a teenager. Most likely, the two have nothing to do with one another; statistical associations are a dime a dozen. In no way does this finding constitute substantial evidence that health problems in infancy cause teenage suicide. But it made a good story.

Let's consider another study: "Is an Educated Wife Hazardous to Your Health?"—the title of a 1984 report in the *American Journal of Epidemiology*. The authors reviewed seventeen hundred couples. Finding an association between men with educated wives and an increased risk of premature death, the researchers confidently concluded that their findings "supported a causal role." In other words, educated wives supposedly are driving these unfortunate men to their graves. Simply on the face of it, one can be pretty certain that the educational level of a man's wife in and of itself does not bring on early death. Men who choose more educated wives probably share a number of other similarities with their peers, any one of which may be the actual culprit. It's another case of seeing cause and effect in a mere association.

The difference between correlation and cause often is downplayed intentionally. Treating them as though they are one and the same is in the interest of researchers as well as the media. It makes research findings appear much more definitive than they actually are.

Back in the last century "watering down the milk" was a common practice employed to squeeze out more profit. This led Henry David Thoreau to the following observation: "Some circumstantial evidence is very strong, as when you find a trout in the milk." Finding an association between two things (say, for example, a particular disease and a certain eating practice) is not the same as finding a trout in the milk. An association between two things merely tells us that one could possibly cause the other. It does not prove it.

The International "Gong Show"

Playing up the differences between rates of disease in various countries is a favorite health hype ploy. Realistically, these differences don't prove much of anything. Epidemiologists call conclusions drawn from such comparisons "ecological fallacies." For example, much has been made of the fact that countries where large amounts of fat are eaten show higher rates of breast cancer than those consuming less fat. This has been cited as proof that high-fat diets cause breast cancer. But if you think about it for a moment, this is not a very convincing line of reasoning. When countries are divided according to how much fat is eaten, you end up with developed countries versus underdeveloped countries. Consider for a moment other things that differentiate these two groups of countries, any one of which might cause breast cancer: for example, pollution, stress, or caloric intake. We just don't know.

Take another example. Japanese men (living in Japan) smoke a lot, and they also have one of the lowest rates of heart disease anywhere in the industrialized world. So, are we to conclude that smoking prevents heart disease? Of course not. These are simply two separate findings that most likely have no bearing on one another.

A group of British epidemiologists, reporting in 1979 in the journal

Lancet, have turned up a strong inverse correlation between national wine consumption and death from coronary heart disease. The more wine consumed in a country, the lower the rate of heart disease. The graphic presentation is quite striking, depicting a descending line for heart deaths from a high point represented by the low wine-consuming countries (such as Finland, the United States, Australia, and New Zealand) to a low point for heart disease represented by the highest wine-consuming countries (such as Italy, Switzerland, and France). As intriguing as this correlation is, once again it is only an association. It proves nothing! When there is no correlation between two things, one cannot be the cause of the other. When there is a correlation, one thing may or may not cause the other.

So, how do we get out of this quandary? How do we advance from correlation to cause? The answer is slowly, through the gradual accumulation of evidence until we draw close to establishing a causal connection. We go from "maybe" to "almost certainly." Granted, it's not completely satisfactory, but it's all we have.

Let's consider, for example, smoking and its relationship to cancer of the lung. In November 1986, E. Cyler Hammond died. You will not likely recognize his name. For over thirty years, he was the chief epidemiologist for the American Cancer Society. His study of 188,000 men published in 1952 first established the strong association between smoking and lung cancer. A four-pack-a-day smoker himself, Hammond kicked the habit as he accumulated his evidence.

The association between smoking and lung cancer is dose-related. The more you smoke, the greater the risk. Heavy smokers have a risk twenty times as great as nonsmokers of contracting lung cancer. Nine out of ten people with lung cancer are smokers. Smoke contains hundreds of carcinogens. Nonsmokers who live with heavy smokers and thereby passively inhale smoke have higher rates of lung cancer.

These multiple associations and the fact that smoke contains numerous proven carcinogens which it carries into direct contact with the surfaces where lung cancer develops come about as close to causal proof as we get in medical matters.

Based on this evidence, millions of Americans have given up smoking. Regardless of clever denials by the tobacco companies, the case against smoking is a strong case, considerably stronger than that for a host of other risk factors. It is based on massive evidence accumulated over years, which is likely to convince any prudent person of the causal relationship between smoking and lung cancer. Smoking serves, however, as a sober reminder of just how difficult it is to establish medical facts.

Both Sides of the Picture

Medical studies have trouble pursuing two things at once. They are usually narrowly framed. More often than not, a study of health risks does not consider possible benefits, whereas the opposite is true in studies of health benefits; possible risks receive little attention. The truth of the matter is that many risks have some benefits, and many beneficial health practices carry some degree of risk. You cannot count on medical studies to add up the costs and the benefits. You are usually left to do this for yourself.

For illustration purposes, let's look at the practice of jogging. As an aerobic exercise, jogging is widely advocated to prevent heart disease. Books extolling its health-promoting virtues are perennial best-sellers; and, in recent years, sales of assorted running gear have climbed dramatically. Nevertheless, jogging is not entirely good for you. Many people understandably do not fare well, pounding their joints against the pavement day after day. For them, injury to vulnerable joints more than offsets any heart-health advantage, and orthopedic problems are just some of the potential pitfalls.

Each year, a few (and I emphasize *few*) unfortunate souls drop dead in the middle of a jog. Dr. Paul Thompson, in a study of Rhode Island joggers, found one death per year for every 7,620 joggers, a figure "seven times higher than the estimated death rate from coronary heart disease during more sedentary activities in Rhode Island." Other risks include being hit by passing automobiles and motorcycles, carbon monoxide intoxication (if you happen to run in an automobile-congested area), altercations with neighborhood dogs, and overexposure to heat and cold. If you are a woman you have the added dangers of osteoporosis and bone fractures and infertility (temporary).

Anyone still for jogging? Even Dr. Kenneth Cooper, the Dallas physician who started it all with his best-selling book *Aerobics*, has tempered his unbridled enthusiasm. This is because of his own firsthand experience with bone fractures and painful heel bruises. He talks about the costs of too much jogging: "I've changed my mind," he said, "I'm running *less* and performing better. If you run more than 15 miles a week, it's for something other than aerobic fitness."

Similarly, a survey of aerobic instructors reported in the August 1986 British *Vogue* showed that 75 percent had either sustained or aggravated an injury through their exercising. Many of these injuries were due to the impact of landing on hard floors.

So, should everyone stop jogging or doing aerobics? It's a matter of trade-offs. If you jog as a *health measure,* you should be sure the benefits outweigh the risks for you. Some people are especially prone to injuries from jogging; people who are obese, for example, as well as those who are extremely bowlegged or who pronate excessively when they run. These individuals might well be advised to select a low-impact exercise such as bicycling, swimming, or skating.

This same line of thinking applies to a host of other "wellness" prescriptions. Too much of what is good for you has a nasty habit of becoming bad for you. Calcium is good for you, but not if you take too much. Why? Because it takes the iron out of your body. Similarly, the current dietary darling, bran, while allegedly curing a host of things that ail you, can rob your body of essential minerals if taken in excess. What about vitamin B6—is it good for you? Sure, but only so much. If you overdo it with megadoses, you get nerve damage! Feet and hands become numb, and you start to stumble when you walk. Fortunately, the damage is not permanent.

One of the latest fads is omega-3 fatty acids. Supposedly, this is the ingredient in fish oil that protects Eskimos (despite their fat-rich diets) from heart attacks. Can you get too much? Yes, because along with excessive amounts of omega-3 you get loads of fat, extra calories, and sometimes too much of vitamins A and D—vitamins that, despite all the good they do, can do real harm when overdone.

Recently I read a report of a thirty-eight-year-old man who mysteriously began to have weakness in his left hand with muscle wasting. As it turned out, he had been pursuing an aggressive program of push-ups on a hard floor, and it was too much. The sustained pressure on his left palm (it wasn't clear why only the left) just at the wrist junction was compressing his median nerve and causing what is known in medical parlance as the "carpel tunnel syndrome." After laying off the push-ups for three months, the man had a full return of strength in his left hand.

Many beneficial health practices carry certain costs, particularly when they are overdone. What does overdone mean? That depends on your particular situation. For example, if you are a woman with troublesome joints but have none of the major risk factors for heart disease and no family history of it, jogging is not a great health idea for you. In contrast, if you are a man from a family in which all the men develop heart disease at a relatively early age, you may choose to jog despite a few orthopedic symptoms. It's a matter of trying to weigh the benefits against the costs as they relate specifically to you.

In a 1987 *Los Angeles Times* article by Robert Cooke, Professor Paul Saltman, a respected biochemist and nutrition researcher at the University of California at San Diego, related the following story about Bill Walton, the professional basketball player. If you have followed Walton's career, you know he has had almost continuous problems with bone fractures and slow healing. During a sports medicine clinic, Walton's doctor was flashing radiographic pictures of the player's ankle, which had not healed in eight weeks. Professor Saltman was aware of Walton's preference for a strict vegetarian diet. He asked if this was still the case. The doctor looked puzzled: "What difference does that make?" As it turned out, quite a bit.

Walton was brought in for an analysis of trace elements in his body. The results showed that he had "zero manganese, half the normal zinc, and half the copper." It was assumed that Walton's commitment to his brand of vegetarianism had resulted in these mineral deficiencies. The manganese deficiency alone could well have accounted for a predisposition to fractures and poor healing. With proper mineral replacement, the immediate problem was resolved. "We made him a supplement," Saltman said, "and within six weeks he was back on the floor playing." Bill Walton's diet may have made him feel good and perhaps was healthy for him in many ways, but it also created a predisposition to bone fractures. Given his particular profession, that was a serious risk.

Health benefits and risks often go together. Studies and reports about them often focus on only one of these aspects. You need to keep both in mind.

The Problem of Being Unique

Medical studies have a second serious shortcoming in their difficulty in coming to grips with our uniqueness. In fact, they are diligently designed to eliminate individual variations, insuring that the results will be representative. Groups are compared and average findings tabulated, so the outcomes do not accurately portray any single individual. They are not about Brad Turner, a forty-year-old auto mechanic, married for the second time, with two teenage children, and living in Gilroy, California; but rather about twenty-five white, middle-aged men living in a large northeastern city.

Whoever you are, if you are not one of "these," the study, by design, has limited relevance to you because it was conducted on people who may differ significantly from you. This restriction is easily forgotten by many medical researchers, especially when the microphone is in front of them and they are asked to discuss the importance of their findings. It's a restriction of which most media people are not even aware.

Let's relate this to the famous investigation of heart disease, the Framingham study. The subjects all came from a little New England town of twenty-eight thousand people. They were largely white, middle-class, church-going, nondivorcing people who stayed put. After almost thirty years, the researchers have been able to keep up with 80 percent of the subjects who are still living!

The people of Framingham are distinctive in yet another way: their rate of heart disease has been one-third lower than predicted. Clearly, this was a study of an unusual population. The findings (widely disseminated as national guidelines for heart-healthy living), strictly speaking, apply only to the people of Framingham: they may be far less applicable to other individuals who differ from them in various ways.

One good example comes to mind. It is fairly well established that the coronary risk factors established in the Framingham study do not hold up for older people, over the age of sixty-five. If you make it to that age, smoking, high serum cholesterol, and high blood pressure aren't associated with a greater risk for heart disease. A puzzling finding since most deaths from coronary heart disease occur among the elderly. No one has satisfactorily explained this discrepancy as yet.

The journey from medical studies to individual application is fraught with difficulties. It's a major stumbling block for people interested in taking action to further their own health. In his 1969 book *Biochemical Individuality*, Roger Williams explained how biochemical individuality is at the root of the problem. For example, consider the physiological effects of alcohol. If you selected one thousand people, permitted them to drink alcohol, and then tested them for sobriety, you would find some striking differences. When their blood alcohol level had reached 0.05 percent, approximately one hundred people out of the one thousand would show signs of being drunk. But seventy people would be stone sober, even after their blood alcohol had reached 0.40, a level eight times greater! The rest would fall somewhere in between. It's easy to see how averages can be quite misleading, because few of us are average. A reasonable safe alcohol level for one person will be far off the mark for another.

Individual differences complicate medical treatment. The problem of selecting a cancer chemotherapy agent is one example. Much of cancer therapeutics has been guesswork, with chemotherapy based largely on studies of patients with similar kinds of tumors. Their average responses would be used to select the cancer agent for your treatment. Once treatment has started, you would likely experience a number of untoward side effects: your hair might fall out, you might become nauseated and experience pain. Worst of all, if the treatment failed you would have to return to square one and start over. Again, your cancer doctor would base the selection on previous medical studies without any way of individualizing your particular treatment.

The problem is similar to translating the results of a medical study like Framingham into individual health prescriptions. It is very much a hit-or-miss proposition. Although large-scale medical studies generate valuable information, as individuals we cannot be certain it applies to us. This is unfortunate because, as we learn more about biological differences, the need for individualized treatment becomes glaringly obvious.

This is well illustrated by important changes now taking place in the selection of cancer chemotherapy, with the "clonogenic assay." An extremely practical technique for individualizing cancer chemotherapy, it represents a major advance in this field. Instead of basing a person's treatment on the treatment outcomes of others with similar cancer, the clonogenic assay uses cells biopsied from a person's own tumor. Malignant cells are removed from the tumor and then grown on laboratory culture plates where they are exposed to several cancer-fighting agents. Through the use of a videomicroscope to follow the amount of malignant cell growth, within a few days the agent that best retards the cancer's growth is identified. In this way the patient's treatment is custom-designed for the specific characteristics of his or her own cancer.

This is the kind of approach we need for working out sound individual health programs for ourselves. The problem is, more often than not, that we don't have enough specific information. What we do have comes from those large studies. Health fiction blithely acts as if there is no problem, routinely applying statistical averages to everyone as a matter of course.

Regardless of how the media reports the health news, health hype will continue to thrive, if for no other reason, simply because so much medical information is limited in its applicability to individuals. That's not the media's fault; it's a problem with the available information. Average findings are better than no information at all, but they have serious limitations.

In a moving, personal account in *Discover* (June 1985) entitled, "The Median Isn't the Message," Harvard professor and essayist Stephen Jay Gould discussed the tyranny of averages. In July of 1982 Gould learned he was suffering from abdominal mesothelioma, an uncommon and virulent cancer often related to asbestos exposure. He relates how he immediately plunged into reading about this unwelcome menace to his life. Primary on his mind were his odds for beating it. In a short while he found his answer. "The literature," he said, "couldn't have been more brutally clear: mesothelioma is incurable, with a median mortality of only eight months after discovery." Gould relates how he sat "stunned," realizing then why his physician had discouraged him from reading up on mesothelioma.

After his initial shock subsided, however, he began to think more clearly about his chances. Eventually he began to challenge this bleak prognosis. He figured it this way: certain things about himself could be expected to improve his chances; for example, his never-say-die positive attitude. Moreover, his whole life showed he wasn't average! He reasoned in his own intellectual fashion: "The distribution was, indeed, strongly right skewed, with a long tail (however small) that extended for several years above the eight-month median. I saw no reason why I shouldn't be in that small tail, and I breathed a very long sigh of relief."

Cancer doesn't treat everyone the same. He'd found reasons to believe he would be one of the longer-lived.

As an afternote, I'm glad to report that Stephen Jay Gould was right. Seven years later he authored *Time's Arrow, Time's Cycle*, convincingly demonstrating that averages are not to be taken too seriously.

Points to Remember

1. Don't confuse correlation with cause and effect. Despite what health hype says, they are not the same.

2. Keep in mind the international version of correlation mistaken for cause and effect. For example, people in countries that consume more fat have higher rates of cancer, *thus*, dietary fat causes cancer. (Socrates would not be amused.)

3. Many risks have some benefits, and many beneficial health practices carry some risks.

4. You are biologically unique. This fact gives medical researchers fits. Medical findings—at least most of the ones you hear and read so much about—are averages based on people who may be unlike you in important ways. Health fiction tries to convince us that one size fits all. It's not true.

▸ ▸ ▸ ▸ ▸

In time Cato's own wife and son fell ill with a mysteri-
ous fever, the nature of which cannot be guessed from
the information we have. Cato fed them cabbage.
Tragically, both died. Cato was deeply saddened. But,
typical of the history of health-foodism, this misfortune
did not change Cato's thinking about cabbages. It is
an axiom of the health-food school, through history,
that no dedicated health-foodist is disturbed by mere
fact.

—Ronald M. Deutsch,
*The New Nuts
among the Berries*

▸ ▸ ▸ ▸ ▸ ▸ ▸ ▸

CHAPTER NINE

Health Hype as Evangelism

The claims and the faces may have changed, but health hype has been around for generations. Convinced they have found the key to health and long life (or, at least, believing they can convince others), health evangelists have spread the word, always finding receptive listeners eager to embrace the newest brand of health salvation. Health evangelism of the past shows us some timeless themes of health fiction that never seem to disappear.

"Natural" foods, "health" foods, and life-extending regimens have made the health hype circuit many times, each occurrence with new evangelists and a brand new flock of followers. In this chapter you'll find enough useful information to keep these zealots from pulling the wool over your eyes.

Natural Is Best

"Natural" has been one of health evangelism's most enduring gimmicks. As a health come-on, "go natural" has shown remarkable staying power. Today's emphasis on natural is simply the recycling of a centuries-old idea. When John Denver stands at the railing of a redwood deck overlooking a mountainous expanse bathed in early-morning sunlight and (sitting down to a bowl of Post Natural Raisin Bran) says, "I've always chosen nature's way," we are not seeing the results of new scientific findings. When the wine makers advertise wine as a natural food beverage containing minerals and other vital nutrients, the hard liquor magnates should sit up and take notice. They are facing one of the most effective sales pitches yet devised: natural is best!

Oddly enough (given all the hoopla), "natural" has no legal definition. Marian Burros, food critic for the *New York Times,* has illustrated this with one of America's best-selling packaged cheeses. It's promoted as natural even though it contains artificial coloring and the food additive potassium sorbate. There are many other examples of the bastardization of "natural." The lack of an official definition makes it easy, but does it really matter anyway? Is natural all that it's cracked up to be? No. First of all, there are instances when there's simply no difference between natural and synthetic. Vitamin C is a good example. Despite claims that it's better for you when extracted from natural sources, there's not a shred of evidence that this is true. Vitamin C is vitamin C. Nature makes it. Chemical laboratories make it. It's all the same. With one exception—the price in health food stores is usually exorbitant.

The same can be said for fertilizer. For years, foods grown "organically" (with natural sources of fertilizer) have been touted by health food buffs as superior. Not so. Whether it comes out of a cow or a chemical laboratory, with respect to three essential ingredients— nitrogen, potassium, and phosphorus—fertilizer is fertilizer. Plants don't seem to know the difference between organic or synthetic. If they do, they don't care. The nutrients in food grown with one or the other are the same.

Natural can actually be less healthy. For example, bread without additives lacks calcium propionate. This additive retards mold and the production of aflatoxin, a potent carcinogen. It also provides a safe source of calcium. (The irony is that calcium propionate occurs *naturally* in foods such as Swiss cheese and raisins.)

Perhaps the most damaging case against "natural" is the one made by Dr. Bruce Ames, a professor of biochemistry at the University of California, Berkeley. Dr. Ames has spent much of his professional career tracking down cancer-causing substances. One of the most widely used tests for carcinogens, the Ames Test, is named after him. In September 1983, Dr. Ames's article "Dietary Carcinogens and Anticarcinogens" appeared in the prestigious journal *Science*. Its message was a blow to natural's health mystique. Ames contended that many common foods we eat *naturally* contain carcinogens. Nature (most likely as a survival measure against insects and the like) has endowed many common plants with poisons, natural poisons. They are contained in foods appearing frequently on our dinner tables: black pepper, mushrooms, potatoes, celery, figs, and parsley, to name only a few. In a devastating punch line, Ames claimed that we probably consume ten thousand times as many natural carcinogens as man-made ones! Not that these natural foods are a great risk to our health. They are present only in minute quantities and would likely be hazardous only if consumed in gigantic quantities, far beyond what is in our ordinary diets. Nevertheless, the point is made: natural does not necessarily mean healthy.

Consider the oils most often used in natural foods. Coconut, palm, and palm kernel are three of the most saturated fats available. Although not proven as causative factors in heart disease, these saturated fats do not come highly recommended as healthy food. These same natural saturated oils are used in making nondairy creamers, allegedly as a healthy, low-calorie alternative to milk fat. The truth of the matter is that these oils contain thirty calories per tablespoon—the same as regular cream itself.

Finally, in our look at the myths about natural, we should not overlook honey. For a number of years it has been one of the natural food stars but its celebrity status is undeserved. As a sweetening agent, honey has the same effects as sugar, including fostering dental caries.

"Natural" sounds nice, but it does not carry a guaranteed seal of good health.

The Early Health Evangelists

Some of health hype's favorite themes have been around a long time. They may occasionally undergo "repackaging," but the essence remains the same. In his informative and highly entertaining book *The New Nuts among the Berries*, Ronald M. Deutsch has chronicled the beliefs and practices of health evangelists over the past century. They are not too dissimilar from many of the headlines we read today. The more things change, the more they stay the same.

The names Kellogg and Post are strongly associated with the cereal industry, but few people realize that the founders of these two cereal giants came to this breakfast food almost as an afterthought. Health and wellness were their first loves, and they fought tooth and nail over the exact ingredients.

Dr. John Harvey Kellogg graduated in 1874 from Bellevue Medical College and became editor of *The Health Reformer*. Early on he put his faith in water, considering it the cornerstone of good health—plenty of water in a variety of forms. Copious draughts of water and strawberries were good for high blood pressure. If the pressure was really high, ten to fourteen pounds of grapes (high water content!) was essential if it was to be brought under control.

Kellogg established a health spa—The San—as a way of indoctrinating people with his ideas about health. One of his guests (a well-to-do real estate salesman and blanket manufacturer from Fort Worth, Texas) was named Charles W. Post. Post left The San still ailing but a health enthusiast nonetheless who soon developed his own program. In his book, *The Road to Wellville*, he discussed the health benefits of "natural suggestion." He was a strong believer in bran and didn't take long to develop his first natural bran product, Grape Nuts (an intriguing name selection given his arch rival's strong belief in the healing powers of grapes). The game was afoot. Natural bran cereals from both Kellogg and Post would eventually capture huge markets.

From today's advertisements you would think that the healing power of bran was a recent discovery—nothing could be further from the truth. We aren't hearing anything that Post and Kellogg didn't say a century ago. It's the same bran in different boxes.

Yogurt and the Dangers of Autointoxication

At the turn of the century, when the competition between Kellogg and Post was heating up, a Russian Nobel Prize winner by the name of Elie Metchnikoff decided the answer to long life resided in yogurt. His evidence was based on the mistaken belief that Bulgarians lived longer than other peoples of Europe. Since Bulgarians eat lots of yogurt, Metchnikoff (falling into the old ecological fallacy trap) concluded that yogurt must be the key. He quickly contrived a theory about "autointoxication." As he saw it, protein lying around in a person's intestine putrefies and slowly leads to self-poisoning. The bacteria in yogurt was supposed to attack and neutralize these putrefying proteins, and—presto—life would be extended.

A long line of health evangelists have been influenced by Metchnikoff's half-baked idea, including Jerome Rodale, the founder of *Prevention* magazine; Adelle Davis, the nutrition guru; Linda Clark, a popular health writer; and Dr. Kellogg himself, who eventually came up with an alternative to yogurt.

Kellogg decided that the only truly safe foods for human consumption were *natural* foods: fruits, grains, juicy roots, eggs, milk, and nuts. He was particularly big on nuts. At one time he was involved in a project to plant four hundred square miles of nut trees to revolutionize the American way of eating. But he ran into a small problem—many people lose their teeth as they grow older. This makes eating nuts a difficult chore. Kellogg rose to the occasion by inventing peanut butter.

Few health fads took the country like the chewing treatment of Horace Fletcher. As Harvey Green describes in *Fit for American*, "fletcherizing" became the word of the day. And what was it? Nothing more than the slow, methodical chewing and rechewing of food. Fletcher thought that thorough food chewing was the key to good health, and he converted much of the country to his way of thinking. When he was asked the basis for his belief, he pointed out that when a person chews food long enough, a natural swallow reflex opens up the throat, allowing the food to pass through. For Fletcher this was like a sign from heaven, showing that "fletcherizing" was indeed the proper way to eat. (As you can probably tell, health evangelists seldom allow themselves to get hung up on logic. If they feel it's right, it's right!)

Horace Fletcher's "fabulous" chewing-for-health movement was lauded in major magazines across the country. Even though he was 40 percent overweight, anecdotal accounts of his superior fitness were widely recounted and helped to promote his ideas. John D. Rockefeller was one of millions of his converts, as was Thomas A. Edison. (So was Harvard psychologist William James, at least for a short while. Later he wrote: "I tried Fletcherism for three months. It nearly killed me.") Fletcherizing was even introduced at West Point. Picture those cadets, sitting at attention, chewing their food until it liquified, and then all swallowing in unison.

Fletcher finally died of chronic bronchitis. A health evangelist to the end, he spent the last weeks of his life arguing with Charles W. Post about proper health care. Post described Fletcher's death as a monument to the folly of insufficient roughage. He committed an entire chapter in one of his books to "Horace Fletcher's Fatal Mistake."

But the title "greatest health evangelist of the century" goes to Bernarr Macfadden. From the early 1900s until 1955, Macfadden extolled the virtues of physical fitness along with plenty of sun, fresh air, and hot baths. Good for colds and syphilis! He advocated walking barefoot, which often he did from his home to his office, where he arrived at noon. His diet included no processed white sugar or flour. He was big on deep breathing and natural foods, "complete foods" as he termed them. He believed fresh fruit kept the intestines antiseptic. (Shades of *Fit for Life*.)

As a side business, Bernarr Macfadden built a publishing empire that included *True Story, True Romances, and True Detective*. With the income from his publishing, Macfadden underwrote his own one-man health education road show. Later in his life, he was nominated at the Republican National Convention for the presidency of the United States but was defeated by Alf Landon. In 1940 he won the nomination for U.S. senator from Florida but lost the election.

Macfadden lived to be eighty-seven. No one knows whether or not his longevity had anything to do with the unorthodox assortment of health ideas he practiced and successfully sold to the American public for decades.

Life Extension

Health evangelism is still alive and well today. If you don't think so, spend a little time in your local bookstore perusing the health and fitness offerings. Some of the more successful "pitches" in recent years offer the tantalizing promise of life extension. Supposedly, if you adhere to a certain regimen, usually nutritional, you can extend your life beyond what you could ordinarily expect to live. One of the most popular regimens has been advanced by two authors, Pearson and Shaw, who let us know that they live what they advocate, complete with "muscle-beach" poses. Their book *Life Extension* goes into great detail (a thousand pages worth), advocating megadoses of dozens of nutritional supplements. The book has sold millions of copies, and people who sell the life-extending substances advocated in the book have also done well.

Is there any substantial evidence that it works? Will devotees to life extension be living into their hundreds while the rest of us die off earlier? Dr. Edward L. Schneider, deputy director of the National Institute of Aging, thinks not. Based on an extensive review of medical research, he concluded that there are no proven methods for increasing the human life span. The review was written for the *New England Journal of Medicine* because officials at the National Institute of Aging were "concerned about the false and misleading claims for products that are promoted to extend life span."

"Life extension" might be worth a try (on the outside chance that it works), but only if you don't mind assuming the risks and the costs of taking huge doses of vitamins and minerals. When you consume thousands of times the recommended daily requirements, you are navigating in uncharted waters. Don't be fooled by the idea that they are "only vitamins and minerals." Keep in mind that large doses of vitamins and minerals act like drugs and can have serious side effects. Also, although minerals and vitamins are regulated by the FDA, it's only to insure that they are 98 percent pure. A rate of two percent impurities is not much when these supplements are consumed in tiny amounts, but megadoses are another thing. Two percent impurities become sizable and may well cause serious problems.

Expense is also a consideration. The price of nutritional supplements skyrockets when they are consumed in bulk. Over a lifetime the expense will be substantial. If you adopt "life extension," understand you are putting your money on a long shot. (Remember, it's based on what makes rats live longer.)

Health Food

The promises of better health and longer life are the driving forces behind the meteoric rise of "health food," now well over a billion-dollar-a-year industry. Health food stores are chameleons. They are regulated like food concerns but act like physician-pharmacy combines. If you are a woman whose physician prescribes megadoses of vitamin B-6 for your premenstrual symptoms, and you develop toxic symptoms of weakness and sensory loss in your hands and feet, you have some recourse. You can sue for malpractice! Compare this to the customer in a health food store. The same "drug" can be sold off the shelf as a nutritional supplement. Large doses can be promoted without any warnings and the customer has no recourse if toxic symptoms should develop. The marketplace prevails. Buyer beware!

Herbal teas are a big item in health food stores, promoted as "natural" alternatives to caffeine-laden tea and coffee. Unfortunately, while free from caffeine, these preparations include other less-advertised drugs. Teas from senna leaves can produce diarrhea. Chamomile and yarrow teas have caused severe allergic reactions in people with hayfever. Psychotic reactions have resulted from brewing catnip, nutmeg, and wormwood. Researchers discovered that Health Inca, a tea grown and packaged in Peru and sold in health food stores since 1983, contained cocaine. The tea had been promoted as providing natural stimulation without caffeine!

Supplements

Nutritional supplements have been oversold. I once received in the mail an advertisement for "sports vitamins." The brochure listed a number of sports such as tennis, golf, and swimming (also fishing!). For each sport you could order prepackaged vitamins and minerals, designed specifically for the demands of your particular sport. Books exhorting us to "eat to win" present a similar line of thinking. Apparently there's an eager sporting world out there waiting for the latest dietary breakthrough for gaining "the winning edge." Given the current trend, it would not be surprising to find future dietary schemes for reducing golf strokes or improving one's tennis.

Well-known doctors sometimes get seduced into making overstated claims for nutritional supplements. That was the case involving a Texas-based company known as United Sciences of America (USA, Inc.), according to a 1986 article in the *New England Journal of Medicine*. The company's promotion rhetoric talked about "state-of-the-art nutrition," and its Scientific Advisory Board read like a *Who's Who of Medicine*. It included Baylor University's chancellor and world-renowned heart surgeon, Dr. Michael E. DeBakey, and Harvard's preeminent cardiologist, Dr. Eugene Braunwald.

With the help of promotional pitches from the likes of Joe Montana and Chris Evert, USA, Inc., maintained that its revolutionary formula was born out of necessity. Toxic pollution, stressful life-styles, and the loss of vital nutrients made it essential that everyone should be taking the company's revolutionary, breakthrough formulas (and perhaps selling the same products door to door to others). Actually, the four supplement formulas were similar to hundreds already offered in health food stores.

This is not to say nutritional supplements are never indicated. Persons with deficiency diseases—such as iron-deficiency anemia— require added vitamin or mineral supplements. Due to decreased absorption, older people sometimes need dietary supplements, especially if their diet is not well balanced. Women who are pregnant require up to 10 percent more vitamins and minerals to adequately supply the extra nutritional demands of the fetus. Women on the birth control pill deplete some of the B-complex vitamins, especially folic acid. Supplements are a sound way of correcting such imbalances.

In recent years calcium has become a nutritional darling. Since 1980 there has been a tenfold increase in calcium supplements consumed by Americans. Women have been aggressively pitched on the value of calcium in preventing osteoporosis (a porous bone condition that leaves a person vulnerable to bone fractures and is estimated to affect up to 40 percent of menopausal women). But osteoporosis is not a simple calcium-deficiency disease. It's far more complicated. For those women at highest risk—white, thin-boned, sedentary smokers—taking extra calcium is insufficient without the addition of estrogen. There's considerable evidence that regardless of how much calcium a woman takes, if she doesn't have enough estrogen, the calcium will not be absorbed.

For the rest of us, including men, some extra calcium is not a bad idea, but if we consume it in excess—say more than about three grams a day—we run the risk of upsetting the balance of other essential minerals such as iron, zinc, and phosphorus. For some of us, excessive calcium may cause kidney stones. Also, because calcium is combined variously with carbonate, gluconate, lactate, and citrate, when we go overboard on calcium supplements, we are getting a large amount of other substances, the effects of which are not well understood.

Getting back to health food claims, most of them are pure fiction created by health evangelists and other commercial interests trying to sell their wares. Despite all the hoopla, longer and fuller lives are not guaranteed by frequent visits to health food stores. No matter. Health food most likely has a bright future. There is something irresistibly alluring about the idea of "fixing" ourselves up with a nutritional tune-up.

When I was a kid, if I seemed a little listless or if school wasn't going as well as expected, my father was quick to recommend a "good tonic" to pull me out of it. Reluctantly, under my father's watchful eye, I would gulp down a slug of vile-tasting yellowish syrup every day until the bottle was finished and, presumably, I had a new lease on life.

Preventive maintenance for the body is a good idea, but it usually takes more than popping a few vitamins or chugalugging a bottle of tonic.

The Great American Pastime

Dieting is the great American pastime. More diet books are written than any other form of health book. In 1985 *Dr. Berger's Immune Power Diet* was a runaway national best-seller. The title was well chosen. Immunity was on our minds, since AIDS had made it a national concern. There was only one problem: special diets don't significantly strengthen the body's immune system. *Dr. Berger's Immune Power Diet* (and a host of other books like it) is speculative fiction. In the chapter entitled "Insiders' Immune Power Tips," Dr. Berger recommended *specific* dietary remedies for a host of things that ail us, including heavy metal detoxification, jet lag, drunkenness, and gray hair—all without documentation. As with so many diet books, the absence of any substantial evidence was no barrier to the book's success. The promise of "revitalizing your body's natural defenses" was too appealing.

Quick to capitalize on the book's popularity, Dr. Berger put out a video entitled, "You Are What You Eat." The advertisement featured a Charles Atlas look-alike with the headline "Get Your Immune System in Shape." As a prospective buyer, the reader is told: "You'll learn how to build up your immune system while you lose weight scientifically." Undoubtedly, the video will also rack up strong sales.

Dieting is also an American obsession. At any one time, about one out of three of us is on some kind of diet. Why? Simple: we eat too much. Then we want to take it off, quickly; thus, the perennial popularity of dieting with its yo-yo pattern of weight gain and loss. Women particularly have developed an obsessive preoccupation with "thinness" that goes far beyond reason. While men have greatly contributed to this obsession, it is women who struggle with the consequences.

There is always a ready audience for the newest approach to losing weight. Any diet book that has a catchy presentation has a good chance of being a winner, even if its claims are off the wall.

One intriguing explanation for a guaranteed market for diet books has been advanced by William Bennett and Joel Gurin in their book *The Dieter's Dilemma*. These authors maintain that dieting is doomed to failure. Regardless of the newest dietary twist, after a while it will fail and a new approach will be needed. Enter the newest diet book. The quest is never ending because dieting is not the answer. *Beverly Hills, Scarsdale, Pritikin, Fit for Life, Rotation, The Rice Diet Report, Elizabeth Takes Off*—all of them are off target. *Losing weight and keeping it off is more than a matter of what you eat.*

The way Bennett and Gurin see it, all those "sensible" rules about what you eat are part of an elaborate folklore that dooms the dieter to sure failure. This perspective is not a new one. It is based on a group of assumptions called "setpoint theory." The idea is that within the brain each of us has a control setting for how much weight our body should carry. Bennett and Gurin summarize the problem: "Going on a diet is an attempt to overpower the body's setpoint. It is not a fair contest. The setpoint is a tireless opponent. It is single minded; relentless in making the dieter so miserable that the diet goes by the way side."

Assuming that there is something to this setpoint idea, how does a person best lose weight? Exercise (with reasonable calorie intake) is probably the best single answer. In addition to burning up calories, it seems to turn down the setpoint, so that the body believes it should carry less fat. But exercising does have its limits. Eventually a weight is reached where further loss is hard to achieve. Regardless of the amount of exercise, the person's weight stays the same. The more a person exercises, the more he or she eats. Perhaps it's nature's way of countering our culture's obsessive concern with thinness.

There are no guarantees that setpoint theory is the last word on losing weight, but it's probably a good idea to keep in mind as a foil to the continuing stream of lose-weight-quick diet schemes.

Truths Not to Live By

It's not difficult to understand why late in their life people often become obsessed with ideas about health. A number of famous people have belatedly found the "key" to long life, and they have not been shy in sharing this insight with the rest of the world.

Upton Sinclair, whose book *The Jungle* did much to initiate badly needed reform in the food-processing industry, eventually concluded that food (even when properly processed) was bad for you. For Sinclair, fasting was the key to health. "I would not like to guess," he stated, "just what percentage of dying people in our hospitals might be saved if the doctors could withdraw all food from them." Not too much later, he began energetically promoting I-ON-A-CO, an electrified collar which, it was claimed, cured most illnesses if worn around the neck for as little as fifteen minutes a day.

George Bernard Shaw latched onto vegetarianism (militantly, of course). John Dewey and Aldous Huxley attributed their long lives to an unorthodox system of subtle muscle movements pioneered by an Australian named Frederick Alexander. Late in her life, Eleanor Roosevelt found the answer to health in certain foodist ideas.

Two-time Nobel laureate Linus Pauling ranks high as one of the world's greatest chemists, but he may well be best remembered as the man who loved vitamin C. He knows as much about the biochemistry of vitamin C as anyone around. His unswerving belief in its healing powers, however, is another thing. Francis Crick, the man who won the race against Pauling to define DNA, said this of him: "Linus isn't always right, but when he is, he's brilliant." He's probably not right about vitamin C.

Pauling believes that vitamin C cures the common cold and retards the growth of cancer. He has put a lot of effort into telling the world about it. (And he practices what he preaches. Reportedly he has taken as much as 18,000 milligrams of vitamin C a day!) There is little doubt that he is one of the most successful "ad men" around. (If all the people who have profited from the manufacture, distribution, and sale of vitamin C were required to pay Pauling for his promotional efforts, no doubt he would be fabulously wealthy.)

Linus Pauling is a modern health evangelist, albeit one with a few more credentials than most of his predecessors. Despite his protests, study after study has failed to confirm his convictions about vitamin C. Undaunted, he continues his crusade, helping to keep vitamin C in the top spot as the most widely used supplement, consumed regularly by fully one-third of the American population.

The Los Angeles Times reported that when Mayor Tom Bradley catches a cold, he tries to fight it off by taking vitamin C. But according to his spokesmen, the mayor (like tens of millions of other Americans) doesn't get much relief from this vitamin therapy. Tons of vitamin C are consumed annually in this country, much of it (one has to assume) disappearing into the sewers as it exceeds the kidneys' threshold and passes from the bodies of the committed.

Luckily, vitamin C is a relatively innocuous substance. And it is cheap. While it may not be accomplishing monumental good, as far as we know—apart from occasional "heartburn" and, with larger doses, a touch of diarrhea—it is not causing most of us a lot of harm. For a few people, however, there can be more serious problems. Large amounts of vitamin C may precipitate gout attacks in predisposed individuals. Those who suffer from the rare congenital enzyme deficiency G6-PD may have episodes of anemia, and the newborn child of a pregnant woman who has taken megadoses of vitamin C may develop scurvy.

The great national vitamin C experiment will likely go down more as a tribute to the salesmanship of a true believer rather than to the scientific acumen of a Nobel Prize–winning biochemist. Overall, little gained and little lost.

There is a moral to all this: Beware of old men (and women) who preach the truth about health and long life. Accomplishments made in other areas of life (impressive as they may be) are not necessarily good credentials for expertise in matters of health.

From "Natural" to Snake Oil

There is a line, sometimes difficult to discern, where the exaggerations of health fiction become the flagrant lies of the huckster. Unscrupulous quacks, looking for the fast buck, knowingly contrive trumped-up health schemes.

In his book *Medical Messiahs,* James Harvey Young relates the story of a seedy pioneer of radio promotion earlier in this century, Dr. John R. Brinkley. Brinkley built one of the nation's most powerful radio transmitters, station KFKB in Kansas City. Between offerings of country music, fundamentalist sermons, and market reports, Dr. Brinkley talked into a gold-plated microphone about "Rejuvenation," a cure for all males who had lost their manliness. The treatment consisted of surgically implanting sliced goat gonads into the "inadequate" man's scrotum. As an added personal touch, each patient was permitted to select his own donor goat from Dr. Brinkley's private herd! The procedure was guaranteed to rejuvenate the patient just like it had "Ezra Hopkins of Possum Point, Missouri."

Health quackery is timeless. There will always be Dr. Brinkleys. The pitch will vary, but the intent will be the same: to make a buck off a bogus treatment offered as a cure for misery.

A perennial natural approach is the water cure. Today's impressive sales of bottled water are reflective of a long tradition. Water of all kinds has been claimed a curative of various diseases. One of the more ingenious, entrepreneurial versions (popular in the 1920s) was "Zola, the Wonder Water." When the postage cost become prohibitive, the originator hit upon the idea of *dehydrating* the water. That's right, dehydrated water! For one dollar, the lucky buyer received a powder marked "concentrated." When forty gallons of water were added, the buyer had an abundant supply of the "best of life-giving beverages."

At first it's difficult to understand how rational people fall prey so easily to quack remedies, especially when the proffered concoctions are so blatantly bogus. But consider for a moment the situation faced by millions of individuals who suffer from some form of chronic disease for which there is no bona fide cure. These people who day after day find no relief from their suffering are ideal prey for hucksters with their false promises of restored health. Late in 1987 two Los Angeles–area companies (Ancient Gold of Van Nuys and Miracles in Motion of Universal City) were charged in a superior court civil lawsuit with fraudulently selling cow's milk as a remedy for AIDS. The companies were accused of bilking desperate people by peddling colostrum (the first milk from cows that have just given birth) as a cure. Tiny bottles of colostrum were sold for thirty dollars each. The *Los Angeles Times* (December 5, 1987) reported that, according to State Attorney General John Van de Kamp, the sellers recommended that users take two bottles a week for the rest of their lives.

People with terminal diseases are particularly susceptible to health quackery. Not so surprisingly even the most sophisticated, in death's shadow, become receptive to bogus treatments. When traditional methods have been exhausted, they grow desperate, and the market is quick to respond. Witness the oddball books aimed at people at high risk for AIDS, pitching new ways of strengthening the immune system. Ludicrous diets and stress-reduction programs are touted as keys to prevention.

Recently an announcement came across my desk that turned out to be a chain letter in disguise. Instead of mailing the usual type of letter, however, you were supposed to mail out material on AIDS for which people sent money. The pyramiding idea was the same. Your name kept getting added to lists, and you made money each time it did. The tie-in to AIDS was added to entice people to keep the letter going, because it was for "a worthy cause." Anything to make a buck.

Since 1951 Dr. Ana Aslan, a Rumanian physician, has been rejuvenating elderly people with a drug called "Gerovital." Its major ingredient is novocaine, an anesthetic agent. Despite scientific reviews showing no positive benefit, each year thousands of people flock to Rumania to receive this therapy. Included among the pilgrims have been such illustrious names as Charles de Gaulle, Somerset Maugham, and Konrad Adenauer. (The only real benefit appears to be the fortune amassed by Dr. Aslan.)

Medical quackery doesn't always take place on such a grand scale. More often it involves individual patients frantically searching for an answer when scientific medicine has none. In October of 1985, Dr. Bruce Halstead, age sixty-five, was convicted in the Los Angeles Superior Court of twenty-four counts of cancer fraud and grand theft. He was sentenced to eight years in prison. As described by the prosecuting deputy district attorney, Halstead, a licensed physician, had sold "swamp water to desperately ill cancer patient victims" for $150 a liter. When analyzed, the substance, known as ADS, was found to consist of 99.4 percent water, the remainder being a murky, brown sludge of coliform bacteria. Acting in his own defense, Dr. Halstead (an early champion of laetrile) portrayed himself as an eclectic, holistic practitioner who gave his patients a "nutritional supplement" to benefit their health.

Perhaps the most amazing aspects of this trial were the witnesses called by Dr. Halstead in his defense. Even after being told of the worthlessness of his treatment, they adamantly supported him. Melodee Wolf (whose six-year-old daughter eventually died of cancer) testified that the doctor "offered me hope because he was willing to at least help."

For every convicted charlatan, there are hundreds that go unidentified. The greatest danger is that they will divert people from more effective therapies; or, when none exist, that they will falsely "push" treatments that make patients sicker and even hasten their deaths.

Points to Remember

1. Health evangelism is alive and well. Don't let its new staging and costumes fool you. Today's versions are no less outrageous than those in the past.

2. Despite all you hear, "natural" is not necessarily best. (If you have difficulty accepting this, think of poisonous mushrooms growing in the wild.)

3. Recommendations for "life extensions" are pure speculation. No one knows. (In fact no one can say for certain that life-extension recipes won't take years *off* your life!)

4. Think of "Health Foods" as a designer label. It sells products that may or may not be healthier. One thing is certain, health foods are more expensive.

5. For the long haul, *diets don't work*. If you are looking to lose weight, go slow. Eating reasonably and exercising is probably your best bet.

6. Don't automatically trust what an aging luminary says about health and long life. If what he or she is offering is expensive and there is no proof of its effectiveness, quickly walk away.

7. When you are hurting is when you are most vulnerable to being taken by a medical huckster, so be on your guard. Remember that even though you may be hurting and nothing has worked, a new "treatment" that makes things worse is not a good deal.

▸ ▸ ▸ ▸ ▸

I think it has become impossible for Americans to keep
their health IQ updated. We are suffering from an
information glut, research overload. But worse, we
have accumulated a midriff bulge of confusing and
contradictory health advice.

—Ellen Goodman,
"This Midriff Bulge of Health
Advice Leads to Indigestion"

CHAPTER TEN

‣ ‣ ‣ ‣ ‣ ‣ ‣ ‣

Health in Perspective

There's nothing wrong with wanting to live a long and healthy life, but no matter how much fiber we eat or how little cholesterol we consume—no matter *what* we do or don't do—we all will die eventually. It's important to keep healthy living in perspective.

This chapter discusses some aspects of a long, healthy, *happy* life that health hype often fails to mention.

Hypeing Life-style

Life-style has been number one on the health hype charts for several years and still shows no sign of losing its top billing. We are told that it's the key to good health. If we would only change the ways we work, love, and play, disease could be vanquished. Eat right (low fat, low calorie, high fiber), exercise regularly, keep the stress to a dull roar, have some friends, get enough sleep, and take "life-extending" vitamin supplements—and health and long life will be ours.

It is a seductive idea—that we can control our health through the way we live. It puts us firmly in charge of our own destinies. There's just one problem: it's not the whole truth. Not that there's no truth in it; just less that what is claimed.

If we live past age fifty, the statistical probabilities of *how* we will die are fairly clear. Most of us will be taken down by either cancer or heart disease, and that's regardless of what we eat or how much we exercise. There is no way of getting around the statistics: 100 percent of us die. To date, no one has managed to escape this final common pathway.

Adelle Davis preached that disease could be cured and even prevented by proper nutrition including raw milk, yogurt, whole-grain bread, and other natural foods fortified with extensive vitamin supplements and free of preservatives and additives. Much to her own surprise, she died of bone marrow cancer, the kind of disease her *natural* regimen was designed to ward off. Nathan Pritikin made millions espousing a rigid, low-fat diet in conjunction with exercise as the formula for wellness. At age sixty-nine he took his own life, depressed and sickened by his advancing leukemia. At some point, life runs out on all of us, regardless of our favorite health regimens.

Health hype has a short memory. It has no awareness of how health beliefs come and go in a recurring pattern; what's being said today is all there is. History shows us otherwise.

At any given time, one of three or four basic health factors gets top billing. People come to believe that there's one main key to health. After a while (sometimes a number of years) the newness wears off; what was held to be the most important factor in health begins to fall in the ratings and is replaced by something else. So, "going to see your doctor" gives way to "environmental" concerns, which in turn is replaced by "life-style" factors, then genetics. Having come full circle, the cycle starts again.

This recurrent pattern has an interesting political connection. In more conservative times (like now), life-style aspects of health are emphasized. Health is portrayed as being largely within an individual's control. The emphasis is placed on living right to stay well. In contrast, during more liberal periods the spotlight is taken off the individual. Sickness is viewed more as the result of a bad social and physical environment or inadequate health care. All these things fall outside the individual's control. Government action is required to make people healthy again.

Presently we are at a point in the health belief cycle where life-style is *it*. Health hype is reluctant to let other factors share the spotlight. But don't let this fool you. It doesn't mean that these other factors don't exert powerful effects on our health. And it doesn't change the fact that there are limits to what we can do for our health by changing the way we live.

Limits to Life-style

Writing in the *British Medical Journal*, Geoffrey Rose, a professor of epidemiology at the London School of Hygiene and Tropical Medicine, coined the term "prevention paradox." In short, he claimed that many of the life-style strategies we hear so much about these days confer only modest health benefits on most of us who practice them. He reasoned that when we are dealing with a widespread health risk, *tiny* gains in overall risk reduction will translate into significant health benefits in the population as a whole. But here's the rub: most of us who take up the recommended practice will gain little, if anything. "A measure applied to many," Rose concluded, "will actually benefit few."

The Professor used the Framingham study to illustrate his point. If throughout their adult life (up to age fifty-five), Framingham men had severely restricted their cholesterol intake (thereby reducing their serum cholesterol levels by 10 percent), one out of fifty men would have avoided a heart attack. This means that forty-nine out of fifty would have eaten a restricted diet every day for forty years with little to show for it.

Changes in the way we live, while important to our health, are simply not as important as health hype would have us believe, and its current focus on life-style unwittingly sets the stage for blaming people who fall ill, holding them responsible for things they realistically do not have control over.

Several years ago, after her own personal experience with breast cancer, Susan Sontag wrote a small book, *Illness As Metaphor*. She described the anger and guilt she felt when people (even her good friends) implied that if only she had taken better care of herself, her cancer would not have happened.

On January 5, 1988, "Pistol" Pete Maravich, college basketball's all-time scoring leader, collapsed and died during a pickup basketball game. Maravich was only forty years old. Upon the news of his death, a flurry of rumors spread concerning the cause—he was back on drugs; he had starting drinking again; his food fanaticism had gotten out of hand. The implication was that something Maravich had done to himself had likely caused his demise. Another self-inflicted, life-style death. A few days later the true cause was discovered at autopsy.

Pete Maravich died of severe heart deterioration resulting from an extremely rare heart defect. He had been born without a left coronary artery. The way he died was directly related to the way he came into the world. It had relatively little to do with the way he had lived.

When life-style's influence on health is overemphasized, it's not long before the appropriateness of providing health care for sick people is questioned. After all, the thinking goes, they have no one to blame but themselves. It's a simplistic view, but often persuasive. Consider the case described in a front-page *Wall Street Journal* article (February 6, 1986) entitled "Scientists Are Learning How Genes Predispose Some to Heart Disease" of two sisters, aged twenty-nine and thirty-one, who developed classic symptoms of coronary artery disease. Their doctors could not believe it. They were too young, and their serum cholesterol was normal. But tests showed that their coronary arteries were clogged. They had serious heart disease, but it was not due to anything they had done. Both of them had been born with a missing protein (apo A-1) whose job it is to collect cholesterol from cells in the body and transport it to the liver for disposal. Without this cholesterol collection service, their bodies had built up life-shortening cholesterol deposits in their coronary arteries. It was out of their control. No amount of dieting would have made a difference.

When you stop to think about it, even smoking is not purely a matter of personal choice. There are genetic predispositions to nicotine addiction that make some of us far more susceptible than others. Additionally, there are powerful commercial interests (aided by our own government's tobacco subsidies) hard at work persuading us to smoke. Lots of things go into a person's getting hooked on cigarettes.

Bad Luck

Years ago when I went off to college, I struck up a friendship with a young woman with whom I had gone to high school. We hadn't known each other very well before college but we became good friends. After her first year, she returned home, married a high school sweetheart, and went on to finish her degree at another college. She became a high school English teacher. I saw her every few years, and she was doing well. She loved her husband and her two children, and she loved her work. She had it together; she kept herself fit and engaged in life energetically. Her husband was building a successful career in the insurance business. One spring morning, their family headed for the beach. At a point in their journey, their automobile was suddenly engulfed in smoke from a nearby marsh fire. They were forced to stop. Visibility was zero. Without warning, a large truck roared down on them from behind, crushing their car and killing my friend along with her husband and two children. It was over—because of bad luck.

Apart from everything else, there's an element of luck involved in how long we live and probably in how healthy we are.

Knowing Our Genes

Winston Churchill was never one for moderation. He was notorious for indulging his appetites. He loved rich foods, good tobacco, expensive liquor, and he eschewed physical activity, as reflected in his excessive weight. Given today's health pronouncements, Churchill, by all rights, should have died long before his time. In fact he lived a highly productive life and had turned ninety years old before he died.

In contrast Arthur Ashe, the U.S. tennis star, scrupulously kept himself trim and in excellent shape. He was active and avoided smoking. Before the age of forty, he had suffered two heart attacks.

What explains this apparent paradox? Genetics. Our biological inheritance predisposes us to certain illnesses and protects us from others. For better or worse, we are not equal genetically. Unfortunately, even in these times of biotechnological wizardry, we do not have precise methods for assessing our genetic predispositions to disease. Our best indicators are found in the medical histories of close relatives: mother, father, grandmothers and grandfathers, brothers and sisters, aunts and uncles. It behooves us to know as much about family diseases as we can. Although their existence or nonexistence is not a perfect measure of our own genes, practically speaking, it is the best indicator we have. By knowing our genes, we can better pinpoint the health risks we should be most concerned about. If close relatives have had trouble with a certain disease, our own chances of getting the disease go up.

Consider obesity, for example. In a study of 540 Danish adults who'd been adopted as infants, American and Danish researchers found that the likelihood of becoming fat was strongly tied to biological parents. Much to the scientists' surprise, the adoptive parents' weight had little bearing on the children's weight when they became adults. Dr. Albert Stunkard of the University of Pennsylvania, the director of this research project, commented on the findings: "Genetic influences have an important role in determining human fatness in adults, whereas the family environment alone has no apparent effect." He went on to point out, however, that this research *does not* show that people with fat parents are definitely destined to become fat. In fact 18 percent of those individuals who had managed to remain thin had biological mothers who were obese. Somehow the way they had lived had helped them overcome their genetic predisposition.

The same principle held true in a University of Utah genetic study of "familial hypercholesterolemia." An analysis of men who carried the gene for this condition showed that on the average they died of heart disease at age 45. However, four men who carried this "bad" gene survived to ages 62, 68, 72, and 81. Again, this suggests that genetic predispositions sometimes can be offset by other facets of a person's life. Genetic density is not completely unyielding.

Health is a mosaic. It is an interplay of various factors. If a person has problematic genes (as reflected in family disease), this should serve as a *special* alert to take whatever precautions are possible in the form of life-style and environmental changes as well as preventive medical care in order to offset the genetic risk.

The World around Us

In his book *The Role of Medicine: Dream, Mirage, or Nemesis?* Sir Thomas McKeown, a noted British epidemiologist, has pointed out that the modern decline in death rates began in about 1850, long before the so-called "miracles of modern medicine." Most of the improvement in life expectancy had already occurred before the advent of antibiotics, open-heart surgery, intensive care units, or even immunizations. It occurred primarily because of environmental changes. Over the past century or so, a number of improvements such as modern sewer systems, water treatment plants, refrigeration, and central heating have helped create a safer living space.

Having arrived at this more hygienic environment in the developed world we now struggle to retain it in the face of growing pollution. Wastes of all kinds are being "swept under the rug," and the clock is ticking. We are confronted with the relentless accumulation of toxic waste materials that threatens the health of generations to come. And no one seems to know what to do about it. Certainly the problem is not within our individual control; any effective solution will require organized effort.

As we move from house to car to work or school and back again, we each inhabit our own *personal environment*. For many of us the automobile has become a second home, providing considerable mobility and privacy but with added risk to our lives. For young adults, the automobile represents by far the greatest threat of premature death. Along with how safely they are driven, the safety design of automobiles becomes a critical health issue. Subtle changes can have profound health effects. Several years ago, when the speed limit on the open highway was reduced from sixty-five to fifty-five miles per hour, few people foresaw the saving of five thousand lives annually.

In a sense, the economy is a powerful, social environmental factor. At Johns Hopkins University, Professor Harvey Brenner has studied health patterns as they relate to American economic cycles over the past century, which he described in his book *Mental Illness and the Economy*. He has shown that a 1 percent rise in the unemployment rate is associated with a notable rise in ill health, premature death, and mental hospitalization. When the economic environment turns sour it brings negative health consequences on a large scale.

The workplace is another important health environment. The number-one cause of time lost from work is not heart disease or cancer but injuries, many of them work related. Roughly four million working years of life are lost each year because of injuries, a number greater than that from heart disease and cancer combined.

Given the current emphasis on life-style, environment remains in the shadows, relatively ignored, but it affects our health just the same. In time it will take its proper turn in the spotlight.

Mind, Body, and Friends

Although there remains somewhat of a mystery as to *how*, there is no question that emotions and mental attitudes strongly influence our health.

A prolonged feeling of hopelessness, for example, is a threat to health. When the stresses and strains of living accumulate, or when an unanticipated loss makes us want to throw in the towel, immunologically our bodies become more susceptible to a variety of diseases from cancer to the common cold. Studies have shown that recently widowed individuals show a temporary compromise in their immunity, supposedly due to a suppression of helper T-cells. These cells play a key role in maintaining the body's resistance.

On the other hand, a positive outlook tends to be health promoting. For example, people who are strongly committed and who actively pursue challenge and change are generally healthier than those who are undecided, passive, and fearful of change. This is not to say that a positive attitude guarantees good health any more than a sense of hopelessness invariably condemns a person to sickness. But our emotions and mental attitudes seem to tip the scales in one direction or the other. Presumably they do so through physiological changes.

The power of the placebo is a well-established medical fact. Hundreds of studies have shown that roughly one-third of patients respond favorably to bogus treatments known to have no medicinal value. The healing power of the mind appears to be closely tied to chemicals in the brain known as endorphins. When the action of endorphins is blocked, positive belief loses its health benefit.

Some of the most important sources of hope and optimism, for most of us, are family and friends. This may explain why supportive personal relationships are so strongly connected with good health. On the average, people with good friends and loving families are far less susceptible to disease than are those who are alone. The odds for good health (especially during particularly stressful times) are stacked against loners.

This is true even in a condition like pregnancy. Pregnant women who are under a lot of stress have far more complications if they are without friends on whom they can depend. In one study complications of pregnancy occurred only one-third as often among women with supportive personal relationships.

Depression is much more common among people who live their lives alone, disconnected from the people around them. Several years ago a group of working-class, British wives were extensively studied. Their lives were difficult; problems such as children in trouble and lack of money were a permanent presence. Many of them, not surprisingly, were found to be seriously depressed. But despite many of the same frustrations, others were immune to depression. The researchers finally determined that the difference had to do with personal relationships. Those women who had at least one close friend in whom they could confide were resistant to depression.

Without a confidant, a woman was ten times more likely to become depressed.

One of the most dramatic examples of the influence of personal relationships on health is "psychosocial dwarfism." This is a rare condition occurring most often in children who grow up in chaotic families. Apparently their social deprivation becomes so great that physical growth is interrupted. The brain's production of growth hormones shuts off in response to the emotional turmoil created by the family situation. When these children are subsequently removed from their homes and placed in more supportive living situations, normal growth resumes.

As adults we can survive living alone, but for most of us, chronic "aloneness" is not particularly good for our health. We are social animals. We do best when meaningfully connected to other people. The medical evidence is compelling—good friends (including family) can be good medicine.

Hospitals, Doctors, and Pills

The health care system makes a major contribution to our health by treating serious injuries and acute diseases. But, like the environment, it also poses certain dangers. The hospital itself is a good example. The person who enters a hospital assumes special risks. In his book *Matters of Life and Death: Risks vs. Benefits of Medical Care*, Eugene Robin describes a study in which 808 consecutive admissions to the medical floor of a teaching hospital were reviewed for complications. The results were not very heartening. One out of every twelve people suffered a potentially life-threatening problem related to hospital treatment. In one out of fifty cases, the complication proved lethal.

One major hospital danger relates to lying in a bed all day. This increases the likelihood of clot formation (especially in the leg veins) and can rapidly become life-threatening if the clot breaks off and is carried to the lungs. This is the reason better hospitals give considerable attention to getting patients up on their feet as soon after surgery as possible.

Another problem arising in hospitals is superimposed infections— infections contracted from the hospital environment itself—as Charles Inlander and E. Weiner document in their book *Take This*

Book to the Hospital with You. They estimate that 5 to 10 percent of hospitalized patients contract hospital infections. Ironically, these infections are some of the most difficult to deal with. "Hospital" organisms, toughened by constant exposure to antibiotics, are capable of causing treatment-resistant infections. They are spread by hospital personnel who fail to wash their hands as they move from one patient to another.

While no one questions the benefits of appropriate hospitalization, the hospital definitely is not a place for procedures that are accomplished equally as well outside. If you are considering hospitalization, get enough facts to assure yourself that the benefits outweigh the risks.

Missing the Point

Health hype encourages us to feverishly work on extending our lives. (The next phase will come with the push for longer life through universal organ replacement.) Considerably less is said about the *quality* of what we are extending. What are a few extra years compared to how a life is lived? The question is seldom raised. Today, there are plenty of people living long, but not-so-full lives. Surely there's more to good health than years.

And there's more to life than good health. There are people who are totally fit yet leading empty lives. On the other hand, there are individuals with debilitating chronic illness who achieve full lives. When you really think about it, good health is a matter of how well you put your life together, not just how fit you are and how long you live.

Where does this leave us? This is how I see it: Much of our knowledge about the health effects of how we live comes from large medical studies. On the average, we are pretty sure that certain practices adopted by large groups of people will show *statistically* significant benefits. The only problem is that there is presently no accurate way of predicting who will benefit and who will not. With respect to the importance of the benefit, those at greatest risk for certain diseases likely have the most to gain from making radical changes in the way they live. For the rest of us who undertake changes in what we eat and how much we exercise, there is probably only a modest health benefit.

In many respects health practices are like a lottery. For those of us with average risks or below, the payoff for meticulous attention to how we live is not particularly impressive. Most of us are involved in a losing proposition when we go overboard depriving ourselves and otherwise making ourselves miserable in a search for good health. But is the alternative to pay no attention? Not necessarily. Consider the following *selective* approach.

First, put lots of energy into things that clearly have high payoff with respect to health. If you smoke, you stop smoking. If you are fifty pounds overweight, you get it down. If a disease is prominent in your family you learn as much as you can about it and what can be done to reduce your risk. If you have a serious disease, you make sure you get the best care possible.

Second, you concentrate the rest of your efforts on *positive* health activities; those things that make you feel alive and good about yourself. You breathe a deep sigh and let go of your "health dread." You accept that there is no way you will ever be able to pay attention to all the factors health hype publicizes. You take consolation in the knowledge that if you stick to those "healthy" activities that you would largely engage in even *without* the promise of longer life and better health, it will be hard to go wrong. Even if it turns out that the health benefits were overstated, the living will have been good anyway. No great loss. Jimmy Buffett said it well: "I'd rather die while I'm living than live while I'm dead." It's a valuable course-correcting thought in these times of "no pain, no gain."

Points to Remember

1. Life-style is not all there is to health, and health is not all there is to life.

2. Environment plays a part. So do personal relationships, genetics, health care, and outlook on life.

3. Health is part luck!

4. Relax. There's nothing to do about it: Death is 100 percent certain.

5. Health's bottom line is putting your life together so that it's satisfying. In this sense, chronic illness is not necessarily incompatible with good health, and fitness and long life do not guarantee it.

▸ ▸ ▸ ▸ ▸

When there's a disagreement between the book and
the body, go with the body. . . . You listen to the
bringers of rules. You consider what they offer. You
test the rules against your truth. You follow them, in
your own way.

—Dr. George Sheehan, *Esquire,* June 1988

▸ ▸ ▸ ▸ ▸ ▸ ▸ ▸ ▸

CHAPTER ELEVEN

Dealing with Health Hype

The next time you feel bombarded with health hype on the newest health risks, diets, exercise regimens, or medical tests, reread this chapter for perspective. Hopefully the following ten guidelines will serve as a source of reassurance against all the health hype hullabaloo. Good luck!

1. Try to keep health risks in perspective.

Living itself is risky. You can die getting in and out of the bathtub. So don't let the newest announced health risk command more of your attention than it deserves. You have to be ready for health hype headlines. Don't have a knee-jerk, panic reaction. Keep your eyes on the bottom line. What is the actual likelihood and seriousness of the risk for *you*? If possible, compare the risk to other risks with which you are more familiar. Just how serious is this condition for which you are said to be at risk? Are the odds more or less than being struck by lightning? . . . killed in an automobile crash? . . . coming down with the flu? What are the *actual* odds of it befalling you?

Don't let relative risk scare you. Even if your risk is ten times greater than someone else's, if the chances of its happening to you are still minuscule, don't lose sleep over it. It's the seriousness of a condition in conjunction with how likely it is to happen to you that determines the actual risk. And actual risk is what you need to consider.

2. Recognize the limitations of medical studies.

A single medical study seldom if ever proves anything. It's only after several studies arrive at the same conclusion that you should begin to take the findings seriously. Furthermore, keep in mind that medical truths are always tentative—they are never established once and for all. They are only approximations arrived at through the gradual accumulation of facts.

Be wary of the temptation to overgeneralize. Although they try, medical researchers typically cannot realistically apply the results of their studies to you with any degree of precision. The people (or laboratory animals!) they study often differ significantly from you. To presume that the results apply equally well to everyone is purely a leap of faith.

3. Understand that beliefs about health (like most other beliefs) are strongly influenced by politics and economics.

Valuable commercial and academic research advantages are tied to health beliefs. In the interest of greater market share, increased number of patients, or additional research funds, results are overstated in order to elicit greater media attention. Health is big business. Recommendations about your health are not always based on what is best for you.

Health beliefs come and go. They are tied to political cycles. As we move from conservative to liberal times, the emphasis shifts from the individual to outside influences beyond the individual's control. Presently life-style is in the winner's circle. The bands are playing and the rockets exploding for what we eat and how much we exercise. Life-style is an important health factor, but right now it's being overplayed. It has its limits.

4. Ask tough questions about "health-promoting" life-style changes.

The bottom line is this: Don't go along with the latest health tip until you have considered the potential dangers as well as the alleged benefits. Remember that your situation is always unique. What may be a considerable risk to your neighbor might be of little consequence for you and vice versa.

The more drastic the recommended life-style change, the tougher you should be with your questions. What's the evidence? Have the studies been carried out on people more or less like yourself or have they been conducted on laboratory cockroaches? What are the real dangers? There's a world of difference in the potential harm involved in taking a few extra vitamins each day versus going on an all-fruit diet for the rest of your life or consuming five hundred times the recommended daily allowance of twenty-five "life-extending" nutritional supplements.

Sizing up health prescriptions is a matter of balancing the significance of risks against the effort it takes to avoid them. Make sure the trade-off is worth your while. Despite what you may have heard (no pain, no gain!), deprivation is not necessarily the key to good health. And it's certainly not much fun unless you happen to be a masochist.

5. Familiarize yourself with your family's medical history in order to better individualize health information for yourself.

One of these days, getting to know your genes may be a matter of having a simple blood test. But not yet. At present the best guide is your family medical history. What do people in your family—particularly parents, grandparents, brothers and sisters—fall victim to in the way of disease? What do they die of? Whatever they have been particularly susceptible to, you likely will be at risk for also, since you share many of the same genes.

If you are a woman, and no one in your family ever dies of heart disease before the age of sixty-five, you may choose not to spend a lot of time reading through the latest spate of heart-health diet books. On the other hand, if you are a man, and the men in your family regularly die of heart disease before they reach their fortieth birthday, it may well be worth your while to spend extra time trying to keep your heart healthy.

6. Identify reliable resources and authorities you can turn to for "second opinions" on matters of health and disease.

One of the best defenses against health hype's exaggerations is to seek out other opinions.

Try to have a "stable" of health resources you can count on: your personal physician, certain health journalists who have earned your respect, health newsletters that specialize in balanced reporting, and consumer health groups. When a health matter is of particular interest to you, consider going to a library or bookstore and researching it yourself.

As for serious medical decisions (such as those that present themselves when a physician recommends major surgery), always seek out a second professional opinion, and if that doesn't clarify things, don't hesitate to get a third. Such decisions are too important to rely on the judgment of one professional. Everyone has a bad day now and then, even doctors.

7. Respect the benefits of health care, but don't lose sight of its potential dangers.

Overall, health care in this country is probably as good as any place on earth. Still, it has its share of risks. Partake of it only when necessary. Inquire about the medications you are prescribed; make certain they are necessary. Enter the hospital only when there is no reasonable alternative. Don't needlessly undergo medical testing, particularly invasive diagnostic testing. Question your physician until you're satisfied that a test is absolutely necessary. Remember, three things can happen as a result of medical testing. Two of them are bad!

If a medical test is appropriate and accurate, it can help provide valuable information. But tests are not always accurate. Sometimes they fail to diagnose a condition you actually have. At other times, they may give false positive results and needlessly lead you into patienthood with its attendant risks.

8. Trust your own sense of well-being as a key guide to what's good for your health.

The efficacy of many health-promotion practices is not well established. If you look hard enough you can find both opposing and supporting evidence. You have to weigh the facts as best you can, trusting your own intuition. This is not so bad. After all, in most ways you know yourself better than any professional ever can. It's your life and your health. So trust your own sense of what's best, especially when medical authorities disagree.

Don't be taken in by today's overemphasis on fitness, beautiful bodies, and long life. It's been said that health is more than the absence of disease. It's also more than being fit, beautiful, and long-lived. Health is putting your life together so it challenges and satisfies you. It's the quality of one's life that matters most. This is not to take anything away from "high-level wellness." But it's not the whole ballgame. The purveyors of health hype never seem to grasp this point.

9. Watch out for health evangelists and health quacks.

Passionate convictions do not guarantee health truths. Be suspicious of "cures" that have no scientific basis. Be more suspicious when it's a "cure" for everything that ails you at a price that will put you in the poorhouse. Be most suspicious when you have a chronic condition. Even though you may feel that anything is better than nothing, be careful. Things can be worse even when they are already bad.

Be ready to walk away when a "wise old man" (or woman, for that matter), previously esteemed in another field of endeavor, proclaims he has discovered the secret to good health. Don't be swayed by the rhetoric, look at the facts. Even if what's recommended is cheap and easy, it may not be worthwhile. Always inquire about the risks involved. Health evangelists routinely fail to mention them.

Enjoy nature but don't fall into the trap of assuming natural is always best.

10. Be moderate.

The idea of living moderately goes back a long way. It's not particularly sexy, but it is sound. Resist radical health-promotion schemes, unless you have good reason to do otherwise. For some, daily "marathon" running and exotic "life-extending" diets may be OK, but for most of us a balanced approach works better than faddish extremes.

At the same time, it's also important to keep this in mind: all things in moderation, *including moderation*. All of us have our personal equivalent of a hot-fudge sundae. From a nutritional perspective it's not a winner: lots of fat and calories; loads of sugar. Even so, every once in a while we need to have one, if for no other reason than that it tastes so good!

REFERENCES

▶ ▶ ▶ ▶ ▶ ▶ ▶

CHAPTER ONE: HEALTH DREAD

Diamond, Harvey, and Marilyn Diamond. *Fit for Life*. New York: Warner Books, 1985.

Goodman, Ellen. "This Midriff Bulge of Health Advice Can Lead to Indigestion." *Los Angeles Times*, September, 1987.

Greenfield, Meg. "Give Me That Old-Time Cholesterol." *Newsweek*, June 25, 1984.

McCormick, James, and Petr Skrabanek. "Coronary Heart Disease Is Not Preventable by Population Interventions." *Lancet* ii: 839–41, 1988.

———. "Holy Dread," *Lancet* ii: 1455–56, 1984.

Samuelson, Robert J. "The Great Cereal Wars." *Newsweek*, September 7, 1987.

"U.S. Ban on Artificial Sweetener Might Be Ended after Two Decades." *New York Times*, May 17, 1989.

Vogt, Thomas. *Making Health Decisions: An Epidemiologist Perspective on Staying Well*. Chicago: Nelson Hall, 1983.

Whelan, Elizabeth M. "Living Longer and Feeling Worse about It." *Wall Street Journal*, January 4, 1984.

CHAPTER TWO: HEALTH HYPE HALL OF FAME

Chapman, J., L. Goerke, W. Dixon, D. Loveland, and E. Phillips. "The Clinical Status of a Population Group in Los Angeles under Observation for Two to Three Years." *American Journal of Public Health* 47, supplement (1957): 33–42.

Dahl, L. "Salt and Hypertension." *American Journal of Clinical Nutrition* 25 (1972): 231.

Hugyahe, P. "Your Heart: A Survival Guide." *Science Digest*, April 1985.

Jacoby, David. "Physical Activity and Longevity of College Alumni." *New England Journal of Medicine* 315 (1986): 399.

Kolata, G. "Heart Panel's Conclusions Questioned." *Science* 227 (1985): 40–41.

Lipid Research Clinics Program. "The Lipid Research Clinics Coronary Primary Prevention Trial Results: I. Reduction in Incidence of Coronary Heart Disease." *Journal of the American Medical Association* 251 (1984): 351–64.

McCarron, D., C. Morris, H. Henry, and J. Stanton. "Blood Pressure and Nutrient Intake in the United States." *Science* 224 (1984): 1392–98.

Malhotra, S. "Epidemiology of Ischaemic Heart Disease and Physical Activity at Work." *British Heart Journal* 29, (1967): 895–905.

Mann, G. V. "Diet-heart: End of an Era." *New England Journal of Medicine* 297 (1977): 644–50.

Moore, Thomas. "The Cholesterol Myth." *The Atlantic* 264 (September 1989): 37–60.

Morris, J., J. Heady, and P. Raffle. "Physique of London Busmen." *Lancet* ii: 569–71, 1956.

Morris, J., J. Heady, P. Raffle, L. Roberts, and J. Parks. "Coronary Heart Disease and Physical Activity of Work." *Lancet* ii: 1053–57, 1111–20, 1953.

Paffenbarger, R., R. Hyde, A. Wing, and H. Chung-Cheng. "Physical Activity, All-Cause Mortality, and Longevity of College Alumni." *New England Journal of Medicine* 314 (1986): 605–13.

"Research News, Value of Low-Sodium Diets Questioned." *Science* 216 (1982): 38–39.

Shapiro, S., E. Weinblatt, C. Frank, and R. Sager. "Incidence of Coronary Heart Disease in a Population Insured for Medical Care (HIP)." *American Journal of Public Health* 59, supplement 2, no. 6 (1969): 1–101.

Solomon, Henry. *The Exercise Myth.* New York: Harcourt Brace Jovanovich, 1984.

Taylor, H., A. Menotti, V. Puddu, M. Monti, and A. Keys. "Five Years of Followup of Railroad Men in Italy." *Circulation* 41–42, supplement 1 (1970): 113–22.

Taylor, William, Theodore Pass, Donald Shepard, and Anthony Komaroff. "Cholesterol Reduction and Life Expectancy." *Annals of Internal Medicine* 106 (1987): 605–14.

Wallis, Claudia. "Hold the Eggs and Butter." *Time,* March 26, 1984.

CHAPTER THREE: THE HEALTH-RISK JUNGLE

Allman, William. "Staying Alive in the 20th Century." *Science 85,* October 1985, 31–41.

Cohen, B., and I. Lee. "A Catalog of Risks." *Health Physics* 36:707–22.

Colburn, Don. "You Bet Your Life, Weighing the Risks in an Age of Uncertainty." *Washington Post* May 21, 1986, Health Section.

Crouch, E., and R. Wilson. *Risk/Benefit Analysis*. Cambridge: Ballinger, 1982.

McNeil, B., S. Parker, H. Sox, Jr., and A. Tversky. "On the Elicitation of Preferences for Alternative Therapies." *New England Journal of Medicine* 306 (1982): 1259–62.

Ruckelshaus, William. "Science, Risk, and Public Policy." *Science* 221 (1983): 1026–28.

Slovic, Paul. "Informing and Educating the Public about Risk." Decision Research Report 85-5, May 1985, Eugene, Oregon.

Urquhart, John, and Klaus Heilmann. *Risk Watch: The Odds of Life*. New York· Fact On File Publications, 1984.

Wilson, R. "Analyzing the Daily Risks of Life." *Technology Review* 81 (1979): 40–46.

CHAPTER FOUR: HEALTH NEWS TANGO

Berkman, Leslie. "Great Earth Settles over Ad Claims." *Los Angeles Times*, January 5, 1988, part 4.

"The Bran Wagon." *Lancet* i: 782–83, 1987.

Eastman, Peggy, former President of the Mid-Atlantic Chapter, American Medical Writers Association. Interview with author, May 10, 1985.

Haggerty, Maryann, and C. Bankhead. "Medicine and the Media: Searching for a Common Ground." *Medical World News*, June 25, 1984.

Jick, H., A. Walker, K. Rothman, et al. "Vaginal Spermicides and Congenital Disorders." *Journal of the American Medical Association* 245 (1981): 1325–32.

Mills, James. "Reporting Provocative Results." *Journal of the American Medical Association* 258 (1987): 3428–29.

Murphy, Brendan. "The War on AIDS: French Announce Dramatic Treatment." *Los Angeles Herald Examiner*, October 30, 1985.

Oakley, G. P. "Spermicides and Birth Defects." *Journal of the American Medical Association* 247 (1982): 2405.

Parachini, Allan. "Lines Form for Wrinkle Treatment." *Los Angeles Times*, January 26, 1988, part 5.

Shilts, Randy. *And the Band Played On: Politics, People, and the AIDS Epidemic*. New York: St. Martin, 1987.

Taylor, Peter. *The Smoke Ring*. New York: Pantheon Books, 1984.

"Tests Cut Toxic Shock Risk." *Medical World News*, January 12, 1987.

"The Vitamin Pushers." *Consumer Reports*, March 1986, pp. 170–75.

Weiss, Jonathan, Charles Ellis, John Headington, Theresa Tincoff, Ted Hamilton, and John Voorhees. "Topical Tretinoin Improves Photo-aged

Skin." *Journal of the American Medical Association* 259 (1988): 527–32.

Williams, P., P. Wood, K. Vranizan, J. Albers, S. Garay, and B. Taylor. "Coffee Intake and Elevated Cholesterol and Apolipoprotein B Levels in Men." *Journal of the American Medical Association* 253 (1985): 1407–11.

Winsten, Jay. "Science and the Media: The Boundaries of Truth." *Health Affairs,* spring 1985, pp. 6–23.

CHAPTER·FIVE: FICKLE MEDICINE

Avorn, J., D. Everett, and S. Weiss. "Increased Antidepressant Use in Patients Prescribed Beta-Blockers." *Journal of the American Medical Association* 255 (1986): 357–60.

Freis, Edward. "Should Mild Hypertension Be Treated?" *New England Journal of Medicine* 307 (1982): 306–9.

Friedman, Emily. "Consumer Group Calls Half of Nation's Cesareans Unnecessary." *Medical World News,* December 28, 1987.

Hershel, J., O. Miettenin, S. Shapiro, G. Lewis, V. Siskind, and D. Slone. "Comprehensive Drug Surveillance." *Journal of the American Medical Association* 213 (1970): 1455.

Pickering, Thomas, G. James, C. Boddie, G. Harshfield, S. Blank, and J. Laragh. "How Common Is White-Coat Hypertension?" *Journal of the American Medical Association* 259 (1988): 225–28.

Ragland, David, and Richard Brand. "Type A Behavior and Mortality from Coronary Heart Disease." *New England Journal of Medicine* 318 (1988): 65–69.

Robin, Eugene D. *Matters of Life and Death: Risks vs. Benefits of Medical Care.* Stanford, Calif.: Stanford Alumni Association, 1984.

Shuchman, Miriam, and Michael Wilkes. "Challenging the Annual Physical." *New York Times Magazine,* September 28, 1986.

Silverman, Milton, and Philip Lee. *Pills, Profits and Politics.* Berkeley: University of California Press, 1974.

Steinbrook, Robert. "Soviet-U.S. Study Rebuts Idea of 'Good' Cholesterol." *Los Angeles Times,* November 18, 1987.

———. "Thousands of Surgeries Called Unnecessary." *Los Angeles Times,* November 13, 1987.

Torrey, E. Fuller. *Surviving Schizophrenia.* New York: Harper & Row, 1983.

Walsh, Maryellen. *Schizophrenia: Straight Talk for Families and Friends.* New York: Morrow, 1985.

CHAPTER SIX: THE PITFALLS OF MEDICAL TESTING

Belsey, Richard, Daniel Baer, and David Sewell. "Laboratory Test Analysis Near the Patient." *Journal of the American Medical Association* 255 (1986): 775–86.

Bogdanich, Walt. "The Pap Test Misses Much Cervical Cancer through Labs' Errors." *Wall Street Journal,* November 2, 1987.

Cleary, P., J. Barry, H. Mayer, A. Brandt, L. Gostin, and H. Fineberg. "Compulsory Premarital Screening for the Human Immunodeficiency Virus." *Journal of the American Medical Association* 258 (1987): 1757–62.

Dalen, James. "Pulmonary Wedge." *Chest,* October 1987.

Fuller, Ethelyn. "Stress Testing: For Whom?" *Patient Care,* April 30, 1986, pp. 52–64.

Levin, Dan. "The Telltale Heart." *Sports Illustrated* 62 (May 20, 1985): 102–14.

"Medical Tests Are Over-Prescribed." *Health Action* (October 1985): 8.

Nishimura, R., M. McGoon, C. Shub, F. Miller, D. Ilstrup, and A. Tajik. "Echocardiographically Documented Mitral-Valve Prolapse: Long Term Follow-up of 237 Patients." *New England Journal of Medicine* 313 (1985): 1305–9.

O'Malley, Michael, and Suzanne Fletcher. "Screening for Breast Cancer with Breast Self-examination." *Journal of the American Medical Association* 257 (1987): 2197–2203.

"Reactive Hypoglycemia: Are You Diagnosing This Uncommon Disorder?" *Data Centrum* 2 (September/October 1985): 13–14.

Robin, Eugene. *Matters of Life and Death: Risks vs. Benefits of Medical Care.* Stanford, Calif.: Stanford Alumni Association, 1984.

Solomon, Henry. *The Exercise Myth.* New York: Harcourt Brace Jovanovich, 1984.

"Tests for Occult Blood." *The Medical Letter* 28 (January 17, 1986): 5–6.

CHAPTER SEVEN: STATISTICAL GAMES HEALTH HYPE PLAYS

Berg, Alfred. "Some Non-Random Views of Statistical Significance." *Journal of Family Practice* 8 (1979): 1011–14.

Cohen, Carl, and Ellen Cohen. "Health Education: Panacea, Pernicious or Pointless?" *New England Journal of Medicine* 299 (1978): 718–20.

Freiman, J. A., T. Chalmers, H. Smith, and R. Kuebler. "The Importance of Beta: The Type II Error and Sample Size in the Design and Interpretation of the Randomized Control Trial." *New England Journal of Medicine* 299 (1978): 690–94.

Gauquelin, Michel. *Birth-Times*. New York: Hill and Wang, 1983.

Gehlbach, Stephen. *Interpreting the Medical Literature: A Clinician's Guide*. Lexington, Collamore Press, 1982.

Hite, Shere. *Women and Love: A Cultural Revolution in Progress*. New York: Alfred Knopf, 1987.

Hook, E. D. "Rates of Chromosome Abnormalities at Different Maternal Ages." *Obstetrics and Gynecology* 58 (1981): 282.

Lever, Janet. "A Sociologist Looks at *Women and Love*." *Playboy*, February 1988.

Moser, Marvin. "Who REALLY Needs Bypass Surgery?" *Rx Being Well*, July/August 1984, pp. 4–5.

Puzo, Daniel. "Raw-Milk Drinkers Reported More at Risk Than Smokers." *Los Angeles Times*, March 31, 1984, part 1.

Sapolsky, Robert. "The Case of the Falling Nightwatchmen." *Discover*, July 1987, pp. 42–45.

Tavris, Carol. "Method Is All but Lost in the Imagery of Social-Science Fiction." *Los Angeles Times*, November 1, 1987, part 5.

Taylor, Robert. "Youth Suicide Prevention." California Department of Mental Health, September 14, 1986.

CHAPTER EIGHT: WHAT MEDICAL STUDIES CAN'T TELL YOU

Breslow, Lester, and J. Enstrom. "Persistence of Health Habits and Their Relationship to Mortality." *Preventive Medicine* 9 (1980): 469–83.

Cooke, Robert. "There's No Such Thing as Junk Food." *Los Angeles Times*, November 19, 1987, part 8.

Gould, Stephen Jay. "The Median Isn't the Message." *Discover*, June 1985, pp. 40–42.

Juarez, L., and E. Barrett-Conner. "Is an Educated Wife Hazardous to Your Health?" *American Journal of Epidemiology* 119 (1984): 244.

Kirk, Neil. "Attitudes to Fitness Now." *Vogue* (London), August 1986, pp. 170, 196.

"New Rules of Exercise." *U.S. News & World Report*, August 11, 1986, pp. 52–56.

Reinhold, Robert. "An Interview with Kenneth Cooper." *New York Times Magazine*, March 29, 1987.

Riegelman, Richard. *Studying a Study and Testing a Test: How to Read the Medical Literature*. Boston: Little, Brown and Company, 1981.

St. Leger, A. Cochrane, and F. Moure. "Factors Associated with Cardiac

Mortality in Developed Countries with Particular Reference to the Consumption of Wine." *Lancet* i: 1017–20, 1979.

Sienko, Dean, Robert Anda, Harry McGee, and Patrick Remington. "Reyes Syndrome and Aspirin." Letter to the Editor, *Journal of the American Medical Association* 258 (1987): 3119.

Thompson, P. D., M. Stern, M. Williams, K. Duncan, W. Haskell, and P. Wood. "Death during Jogging or Running." *Journal of the American Medical Association* 242 (1979): 1265–67.

Williams, Roger. *Biochemical Individuality: The Basis for the Genotrophic Concept*. Austin: University of Texas Press, 1969.

CHAPTER NINE: HEALTH HYPE AS EVANGELISM

Ames, Bruce N. "Dietary Carcinogens and Anticarcinogens." *Science* 221 (1983): 1256–64.

Bennett, William, and J. Gurin. *The Dieter's Dilemma*. New York: Basic Books, 1983.

Berger, Stuart. *Dr. Berger's Immune Power Diet*. New York: New American Library, 1985.

Deutsch, Ronald. *The New Nuts among the Berries*. Palo Alto, Calif.: Bull Publishing, 1977.

Green, Harvey. *Fit for American*. New York: Pantheon Books, 1986.

Kendall, John. "Firms Charged with Selling Milk as AIDS, Cancer Cure." *Los Angeles Times*, December 5, 1987, part 2.

Pearson, Durk, and S. Shaw. *Life Extension*. New York: Warner Books, 1983.

Schneider, Edward, and J. Reed. "Life Extension." *New England Journal of Medicine* 312 (1985): 1159–68.

Stare, Fredrick. "Marketing a Nutritional 'Revolutionary Breakthrough' (Trading On Names)," *New England Journal of Medicine* 315 (1986): 971–73.

Truswell, A. Stewart. "Vitamin C—No Good for the Common Cold." *New England Journal of Medicine* 315 (1986): 709.

Young, James Harvey. *Medical Messiahs: A Social History of Health Quackery in Twentieth-Century America*. Princeton, N.J.: Princeton University Press, 1967.

CHAPTER TEN: HEALTH IN PERSPECTIVE

Bishop, Jerry. "Scientists Are Learning How Genes Predispose Some to Heart Disease." *Wall Street Journal*, February 6, 1986.

Brenner, Harvey. *Mental Illness and the Economy*. Boston: Harvard University Press, 1973.

Brown, G. W., M. N. Bhrolchain, and T. Harris. "Social Class and Psychiatric Disturbance among Women in an Urban Population." *Sociology* 9 (1975).

Hunter, Lisa. *Friends Can Be Good Medicine*. Sacramento: California Department of Mental Health, 1982.

Inlander, Charles, and E. Weiner. *Take This Book to the Hospital with You*. Emmaus, Pa.; Rodale Press, 1985.

Levine, Jon, N. Gordon, and H. Fields. "The Mechanism of Placebo Analgesic." *Lancet* (1978): 654–57.

Lipp, Martin. "'Right' Lifestyle Doesn't Equal a Longer Life." *San Francisco Chronicle*, May 6, 1985.

McKeown, Thomas. *The Role of Medicine: Dream, Mirage, or Nemesis?* Princeton, N.J.: Princeton University Press, 1979.

Powell, G., J. Brasel, and R. Blizzard. "Emotional Deprivation and Growth Retardation Simulating Idiopathic Hypopituitarism." *New England Journal of Medicine* 276 (1967): 1271–78.

Robin, Eugene. *Matters of Life and Death: Risks vs. Benefits of Medical Care*. Stanford, Calif.: Stanford Alumni Association, 1984.

Rose, Geoffrey. "Strategy of Prevention: Lessons from Cardiovascular Disease." *British Medical Journal* 282 (1981): 1847–51.

Sontag, Susan. *Illness As Metaphor*. New York: Random House, 1979.

Stein, M., R. Schiavi, and M. Camerino. "Influence of Brain and Behavior on the Immune System." *Science* 191 (1976): 435–40.

Stunkard, A., T. Sorensen, H. Craig, T. Teasdale, R. Chakraborty, W. Schull, and F. Schulsinger. "An Adoption Study of Human Obesity." *New England Journal of Medicine* 314 (1986): 193–98.

Williams, Roger, Sandra Hasstedt, Dana Wilson, K. Ash, Frank Yanowitz, Gayle Reiber, and Hiroshi Kuida. "Evidence That Men with Familial Hypercholesterolemia Can Avoid Early Coronary Death." *Journal of the American Medical Association* 255 (1986): 219–24.